NURSING THE SPIRIT

Nursing the Spirit

CARE, PUBLIC LIFE, AND THE DIGNITY OF
VULNERABLE STRANGERS

Don Grant

Columbia University Press
New York

Columbia University Press
Publishers Since 1893
New York   Chichester, West Sussex
cup.columbia.edu

Library of Congress Cataloging-in-Publication Data
Names: Grant, Don S., author.
Title: Nursing the spirit : care, public life, and the dignity of
vulnerable strangers / Don Grant.
Description: New York : Columbia University Press, 2023. |
Includes bibliographical references and index.
Identifiers: LCCN 2022043851 (print) | LCCN 2022043852 (ebook) |
ISBN 9780231200509 (hardback) | ISBN 9780231200516 (trade paperback) |
ISBN 9780231553650 (ebook)
Subjects: MESH: Philosophy, Nursing | Spirituality | Nurse's Role
Classification: LCC RT84.5 (print) | LCC RT84.5 (ebook) | NLM WY 86 |
DDC 610.7301—dc23/eng/20230210
LC record available at https://lccn.loc.gov/2022043851
LC ebook record available at https://lccn.loc.gov/2022043852

Cover design: Milenda Nan Ok Lee
Cover image: Hananeko_Studio © Shutterstock

To Tammy, my wife, best friend, and all-time favorite care professional. And to Dad, a wonderful parent who showed me that religion is about more than believing.

CONTENTS

PREFACE ix

Chapter One
Religion and Care of the Stranger   1

Chapter Two
The History of Caritas in Health Care   39

Chapter Three
Craft Versions of Religious Authority   66

Chapter Four
Second-Guessing Talk About Spirituality   90

Chapter Five
Pathways to Spiritual Meaning and Emotional Dead Ends   118

Chapter Six
Styles of Spiritual Care   143

Chapter Seven
Bridging Science and Spirituality Through Storytelling   173

Chapter Eight
Restoring the Sanctity Once Bestowed on Humanity   203

NOTES   221

REFERENCES   227

INDEX   245

PREFACE

For most of human history, care was restricted to family and friends. It was not until the Axial Age (800–200 BCE) that communities first began to recognize all humans, including foreigners, immigrants, enemies, and other strangers, as spiritual beings deserving of protection and nurture. In the years since, however, this fundamental principle of the world religions has increasingly been questioned as societies have modernized and developed care systems grounded in scientific approaches that are indifferent, if not hostile, to the notion that humans possess a transcendent quality. This book seeks to discern the fate of this principle by investigating how an academic medical center's nursing staff variously integrates spirituality into its care work.

In exploring this issue, this study also points to a new understanding of the social significance of religion. Religion is obviously significant to many people at a personal level—at its best, it can offer comfort, guidance, inspiration, hope, and meaning. But when is religion significant beyond the personal lives of individuals—when does it have an effect on societies at large? In the past, scholars have answered this question in one of two ways. The first way is by looking at the influence religious authorities exert over social institutions like governments and schools (Chaves 1994). In this view, we can tell that religion is important in a society when we can see religious authorities shaping how other institutions operate. The second approach is to look not at religious authorities but at individuals as they practice their religion (Ammerman 2013). In this view, we can tell that religion is important in a society when we see people living out their faith in their everyday lives with the support of their "spiritual tribe."

This book offers a third approach that focuses not on religious authorities or religious individuals, but on the principle of *caritas*, which is what the Axial ethic is often referred to in the West. Caritas describes a love, reverence, and care for all people grounded in a belief that every individual has a spiritual dimension of ultimate importance. When we place caritas at the center of our attention, we can see that religion is important in a society when its most vulnerable members are revered through acts of care.

In developing this approach, I draw heavily on the foremost social theorist of the past century—Max Weber. Weber was the first to argue that the religious principle of caritas was at risk in contemporary society (Weber 1958a), and in some of his writings (Weber 1958c, 1978) he also suggested that five key social mechanisms—authority, language, emotions, actions, and narrative—will determine whether values like caritas "stick" in modern settings. To determine if this moral principle can still take hold, therefore, I investigate whether nurses assume responsibility for patients' spiritual care, make spirituality a part of their everyday discourse, feel more authentic when viewing their care in spiritual terms, put spirituality into practice when interacting with patients, and treat spirituality as credible and important in the stories they construct about their work experiences. To the extent that they do, caritas, as a cultural and social phenomenon, can be said to endure.

Determining whether caritas can be transmitted through these mechanisms is especially urgent today. The rise of despotic leaders, divisive and hateful rhetoric, manufactured outrage over critical race theory, indifference to racialized acts of violence, and diatribes against mask mandates suggest that Axial values about honoring and protecting strangers are being rejected and replaced by virulent forms of parochialism. Compounding this problem is the development of biotechnologies and radical medical procedures designed to "improve" humanity, ranging from cloning, cryonics, and gene therapy to nanotechnological implants, stem cell research, and organ transplants. These developments encourage us to approach the human being as a set of physical components to be transformed, optimized, and commodified instead of an intrinsically dignified and worthy spiritual whole (Turner 2017). On top of this is the climate crisis brought on by society's continued burning of fossil fuels, which most immediately impacts the poor but ultimately threatens everyone. Indeed, the chief question before us today is, as Erich Fromm (1963) once suggested, not whether God is dead but whether the sanctity of humanity, if not humanity itself, will soon be.

Readers may want to know who I am and how I became interested in this topic. I am a professor of sociology at the University of Colorado–Boulder, where I am a fellow at the Renewable and Sustainable Energy Institute. I also direct two university-wide certificate programs, one labeled "Care, Health, and Resilience" that prepares students for careers in the helping professions and another labeled "Social Innovation" that equips students to design and execute solutions to some of society's most intractable problems. Although my discipline of sociology covers a wide range of topics, including religion, my formal training in graduate school focused on the more mundane matters of class inequality, political economy, and environmental degradation. Partly for that reason, when I first shared my plan to study nurses' spiritual care with a visiting professor who was familiar with my training and specialized in organizational and environmental disasters, he playfully mocked my interests by tossing a wad of paper at me. But, like many early American sociologists, I was also raised in a family that was religious. And my family was progressive; my dad, for example, was involved in the antiwar and civil rights movements of the 1960s. Partly because of the resistance he experienced from those who believed religion should be an entirely private matter, I have long been interested in the tension between religion and modern public life and whether the two might be reconciled, as was Weber.

I came to study nurses largely by accident. During my first sabbatical, I decided to take a break from crunching social survey data and reflect on where my life was heading by entering a training program for chaplains at a local hospital where I could experience social life and the existential issues it raises up close. After several weeks of fumbling and bumbling my way as a chaplain intern, I came to rely heavily on nurses in figuring out how to approach patients and address their spiritual needs, and I often found nurses' recommendations more helpful than the advice I received in the chaplaincy program. Before finishing my time in the chaplaincy program and returning to my work as professor, I decided to launch a study of nurses' spiritual care and, in so doing, further my budding interest in Weber's writings on the Axial Age.

My engagement with the topic did not stop there, however. Years later I found myself at another university hospital, but this time as a living liver transplant donor to my dad. This experience gave me glimpses into the fate of caritas from the perspective of a patient, and what's more, a patient who was subject to the type of radical biotechnical procedure that some suggest could fundamentally transform human ontology in the future by conceivably upgrading and supplementing the body. This experience made Weber's concern about the survival of caritas even more compelling to me and gave new insight into the precarious place of human qualities like the spiritual in ultramodern care settings.

This book is an outcome of all three of these experiences: as caregiver, scholar, and care recipient. Each of these experiences has informed my understanding of caritas, and each can help shed light on the importance of caritas and its fate in modern society. Accordingly, the book is composed of three interweaving strands about my time as a chaplain intern (in *italics*), my analyses of issues raised by that experience (in regular type), and my observations as a transplant donor (in **bold** type). Braiding materials in this fashion is a technique that many writers use to reveal how seemingly disparate story lines relate to a common theme. My hope is that it will achieve a similar effect in terms of this book's umbrella theme about caritas, illuminating facets of that religious ethic from three contrasting viewpoints. By joining the analytical and personal, I also seek to illustrate how academic research might be humanized, how scholarly questions about care are (or can be) intertwined with the lived experience of giving and receiving of care.

Like the colleague I mentioned previously, some readers who are unfamiliar with existing scholarly discourse on spirituality might instinctively object that the spiritual is too mushy, ephemeral, and idiosyncratic to be worthy of academic inquiry. Some may question whether care of a spiritual variety has any social relevance. And because my experiences as a giver and recipient of care are highly personal, more than a few academic readers may worry that in retelling these experiences I tread the slippery slope of subjectivity.

In response to these concerns, I would stress that the goal here is not to prove that a supernatural realm exists or to endorse any traditions and practices that allegedly tap into it. Nor do I seek to add to the tiresome knockdown arguments of religious and scientific purists. Rather, I am interested in what Marilynne Robinson (2012) and sociologists like Weber say is the first obligation of religion—to value humanity—and whether the Axial idea that all individuals possess a transcendent quality and therefore are worthy of compassion can still be rendered plausible in modern public life. Understood in this light, nurses' spiritual care is a microcosm of the challenges and possibilities of instantiating this ethic in the larger society. As to the dangers of subjectivity, readers will have to judge for themselves whether the text lapses into sentimentality and self-indulgence. My hope, though, is that it will at least suggest how stepping outside the ivory tower and into the realm of care can be a valuable means of understanding the social world and cast additional light on the chapters' analytic themes.

This book's braided strands of material are meant to be read in the order they appear. However, depending on their interests, readers may want to concentrate on some more than others. The analysis strand may be especially relevant to scholars interested in related topics like the porous boundaries between the sacred and the secular and how corporate-sponsored meanings are translated by frontline personnel. The strands reporting my experiences as a chaplain intern and transplant donor may be particularly germane to helping professionals and their clients who want to better understand how this book's chief questions about the survival of caritas are relevant to their experiences or how I became personally interested in those questions. Still, I believe readers will get the most out of the book in reading all three strands because it is only when we relate the study of care to our personal experience of it that we can begin to fully appreciate what is at stake with respect to caritas.

This project benefited from the support of numerous colleagues and collaborators, including Corey Abramson, Al Bergesen, Kelly Besecke, Kraig Beyerlein, Wendy Cadge, Cindy Cain, Mark Chaves, David Cook-Martin, Mathieu Desan, Beth Duckles, Rebecca Erickson, Joelle Fraser, Andrew Greeley, Lisa Ohlen Harris, Sara Horton-Deutsch, Stefanie Mollborn, Alfonso Morales, Calvin Morrill, Kathleen O'Neil, Kelsey Osgood, Rachel Rinaldo,

Jeff Sallaz, Christine Scheik, David Snow, Laura Stephens, Larry Vande-Creek, Iain Wilkinson, and Robert Wuthnow. The Louisville Institute provided financial assistance during the early stages of this work. I am deeply appreciative of Eric Schwartz and others at Columbia University Press for their continued support of my research. I was sustained throughout this project, like so many other challenges, by the love of my family. Special thanks go to the nurses and other hospital staff members for their care and willingness to share their opinions and experiences with me.

NURSING THE SPIRIT

Chapter One

RELIGION AND CARE OF THE STRANGER

I cannot see the doctors, only their shadows beneath the door as they prepare to enter and deliver their decision—a death sentence or permission to go to the next round. I am alone in a room lit by shafts of sun that reveal on the clock opposite me that the time is 6:05 A.M. Stripped down to my socks and underwear, I have been sitting on an aluminum observation table, gripping its edges, and awaiting their arrival.

When they finally open the door, artificial light precedes them, stretching out into this dusky, holding cell of sorts. I squint as the light crosses my face. It then quickly retreats as they make their entrance and the door swings shut behind them. They momentarily disappear in darkness until my eyes adjust.

I first make out their white lab coats and then their facial features. The youngest of them—interns, I presume—are wide-eyed, well groomed, and scarcely able to conceal their fascination. Clutching folders of printouts, they huddle behind their older superior, whom I am meeting for the first time. Like so many others I have encountered at this place, he seems to be scrutinizing my midriff, as if wanting to ask it questions.

Having undergone extensive blood work and other preliminary tests, I am so exhausted at this point from trying to read others' faces and guess their assessments that I do not look into his eyes either. I peer instead over his shoulder at the group of interns, annoyed by their curiosity, wondering how they respond when the verdict is bad, as it often is.

But, to my surprise, the verdict this time is positive.

At first, I do not clearly hear or comprehend what the group's leader is saying to me. But as he continues giving me the results of our tests, it becomes obvious that we have passed them all. "Your liver is a match and you are a suitable donor for your father," he says. "We have scheduled his transplant to begin at midnight."

"You mean in just eighteen hours?" I ask.

"Yes."

I am struck by how matter-of-factly he delivers the news. Maybe it is because living donor liver transplants have become commonplace at this center; it now performs over thirty such procedures a year. Or perhaps he is trying to be reassuring.

Whatever the case may be, no sooner am I relieved to hear we qualified to have the transplant than I start to feel unsettled. It is hard to fathom that a portion of my liver can be cut out and transplanted into my father and what little remains in me will grow back to its original size and shape. I worry that the team's assessment has not been sufficiently thorough and there are complications they are unwilling to acknowledge and maybe incapable of addressing. I am only told that I am qualified for the procedure without being informed about the odds that it will work. I am also told that I will not get to speak with the lead surgeon, Amadeo Marcos, until the day after the procedure. So, I ask his chief assistant, whom the interns are gathered around, what is the most difficult case his team has ever dealt with.

He flashes a grin and replies, "The most difficult involved a transplant recipient with a tattoo of Jesus on his abdomen. He made us swear that we would make Jesus's face look exactly like it did before the surgery. It took us an extra two hours—twenty hours total—but we did it."

I chuckle at the thought of exhausted surgeons having to reset the Son of Man's disjointed nose, lips, and eyes. I then try to imagine what kind of person on the verge of death could make such a request. Perhaps someone who wanted to make sure his admission stamp to heaven would still be valid. Or who was not religious at all but was just into eternity art. There is no telling. Whatever his motives, there was apparently a sublime quality about the tattoo that he wished to preserve and have forever affixed to his being.

I gather from the surgeon's comments that, with most inked-up patients, the transplant team runs roughshod over tattoos, leaving them disfigured, perhaps beyond recognition. But they made an exception for this person and kept his holy inscription intact. What I do not fully understand, though, is why that would require extra time and effort. Wouldn't the surgeons want to realign the skin exactly as before, regardless of whether a patient had a tattoo? Wouldn't they have to for the procedure to be a success? Or are they slapdash butchers racing to process the next slab of meat coming down the conveyer belt?

I would like to know so much more about what we have gotten ourselves into, but we have run out of time and options. The fact is that I never had much time to ask questions. Therefore, I have no real idea how the transplantation procedure actually works, let alone what can be done if they botch the transplant or if the graft does not take. Who will help us pick up the pieces? Obviously, not these meat packers, adorned in their white robes. For them, it's a struggle to just preserve some semblance of the sacred.

I try to stop going further down this rabbit hole by reminding myself how fortunate my dad and I are to qualify for this lifesaving operation. It works for a while, until the chief assistant and his interns give me one last medical gaze and exit the room. I am now supposed to get dressed and fill out additional paperwork two floors below. But I remain seated on the exam table, staring at the clock.

It dawns on me how foolish my family and I were to let our desperate situation, the fact that my dad is too old to have a reasonable chance of getting a "normal" transplant, distract us from learning more about the surgery, its mortality rates, and its possible long-term complications. The day before, a medical social worker quizzed me about my mental and emotional preparedness for the procedure. She quipped that she knew of donors who went into hiding after being told their liver was a match. Her remark did not make sense to me then, but it begins to now. The ceiling vent above seems to grow louder as I reflect on how my dad and I are probably little more than cash cows to this place—half-million cash cows, to be more exact.

I eventually ease myself down from the table and slip into the gown left for me. Tightly holding its rear flaps together, I walk to the exam room door and poke my head out, looking down the corridor for someone, anyone. Several people pass by—a janitor leisurely pushing a mop and bucket, a tech pulling an IV pole with a wobbly rear wheel, and several family members hastily searching for their loved ones' room numbers.

None of their eyes meet mine until a nurse, rooting in her purse, comes down the hall. She pulls out car keys and a pack of Esse cigarettes as she slows to find out what I am doing. She is the first staff worker today to look me directly in the face. I am taken back by this and uncertain how to begin.

I blurt out, "This is quite a center, isn't it? I overheard that the new transplant chief, Dr. Marcos, is really ramping up operations."

"He is ramping things up, all right . . . Look, I hate to say this, but I am sort of in a hurry. Is there something you need or I can help you with?"

"I am not sure. I guess I wanted to know a little more about the risks involved in a living donor liver transplant. Do you know anything about that? If things go wrong during the operation or afterward, can anything be done? Should the surgery fail and things fall apart, will there be someone to help us?"

"Sure as hell not Marcos," she mutters.

Her look quickly softens. "Listen, we will be there with you at every step to make sure you get through this. But if you are having doubts about the operation itself, you probably should consult one of the surgeons, because I have to leave right now."

"That's okay. I just spoke with one of them, the chief assistant . . . Thanks anyway."

As I withdraw back into the exam room, I catch a glimpse of a white-and-pink button pinned to her purse. It reads, "Nurses may not be angels, but they are the next best thing." Not the warm and fuzzy message I was seeking, but it's comforting nonetheless in this otherwise sterile environment.

Human anguish prompts spiritual concerns. It stirs up feelings of insecurity, exposes life's unfairness, and raises troubling questions about the ultimate worth of human lives. Yet the problem of suffering is typically treated by highly bureaucratic and technical systems that can trivialize such spiritual concerns, making them seem quaint, awkward, and retrograde. Scientific medicine is one such system: hospitals rely on bureaucracy and technology, and the hospital nurses who are responsible for most of the interaction with patients are trained in this scientific approach and for the most part not in spiritual care. At the same time, nurses are increasingly asked to care for patients' spiritual well-being—to honor and perhaps expand a sense of purpose and meaning in their lives. How do nurses respond? How, if at all, do these workers who are the "next best thing" to angels integrate spirituality into their science-based work with patients?

This book addresses that question by surveying and interviewing nurses working at one of the largest university hospitals in the southwestern United States (referred to here as University Hospital).[1] As some of the most technologically advanced and bureaucratically intense facilities in the world, hospitals' discoveries and successes have cast doubt on many traditional religious understandings, including the notion that individuals possess a spiritual or godlike quality, because these very successes seem to suggest that reality is wholly material in nature. In response to complaints about their impersonal outlook and nature, academic medical centers have recently promoted a holistic form of care that recognizes patients as biologically, psychologically, socially, and spiritually constituted. In order to legitimize hospitals in the eyes of potential patients, nurses must now try to coordinate science and spirituality. This effort to introduce spirituality into a scientific environment makes public teaching hospitals an ideal setting for determining whether frontline care professionals take spirituality seriously in a context where science is the guiding principle.

Examining this issue provides a window into the fate of humanity's most significant spiritual revolution, what German philosopher Karl Jaspers called the Axial Age (800–200 BCE).[2] During the Axial Age, religions around the world began to turn—as if on a giant global axis—from exclusive concern with one's own local group toward advocacy for the inherent spiritual dignity of all human beings. It was during this period that care for the stranger first became a core religious value.

Scholars have debated whether this transcendent, universal ethic can survive in modern times. Optimists contend that "nothing is ever lost in evolution" and that the axial theme of loving others without distinction is still present today (Bellah 2011; Bellah and Joas 2012; Habermas 2010).

Pessimists argue that religion is inherently parochial and doubt that it ever turned people into unconditional altruists (Haidt 2012) or argue that, if it did, its supernatural beliefs have long since been discredited by science (Dennett 2006; Dawkins 2011).

Neither camp, however, has explored the experiences of caregivers themselves—those who actually do the work of caring for strangers. In modern societies, much of this care has been professionalized: social workers, counselors, teachers, and health care practitioners look after the well-being of the vulnerable in spaces like public hospitals devoted to the "care of strangers" (Rosenberg 1987). What do these workers think about the status of spiritual conceptions of humanity? Do they approach their care work with a sense of reverence for each person's transcendent worth? How do they reconcile a spirit of care with social structures that typically emphasize modern values of objectivity, efficiency, and secularity?

In asking whether nurses working at an academic medical center still render the type of spiritually sensitive care advocated by Axial thinkers, or what in Western society is often called caritas (Jackson 1999), this book also offers a new way to think about religion and its place in public life. Scholars have long argued that as societies modernize, theocracies are dismantled, religion is pushed out of public life, and spirituality begins to be seen as a private matter that is pursued only with family members and one's religious community (Wilson 1976; Chaves 1994). Others have disagreed, suggesting that most people carry their spiritual lives with them beyond places of worship into online communities, dinner groups, classes, workshops, retreats, and other ordinary spaces where they can experience the sacred in the company of those with a similar spiritual identity and outlook (Ammerman 2013). Each of these perspectives offers a different view of the notion of "public religion." In the first view, religion is public when religious leaders have considerable influence over powerful social institutions such as governments and workplaces. In the second, religion is public when religious individuals bring their spiritual sensibilities into their everyday lives outside religion.

This book takes a different approach. Religion is public, I argue, when human beings are revered through acts of care—including those outside one's group and in settings that may otherwise seem indifferent or hostile to the sacred. Religion's public presence in a society, in other words, can be measured by its care for the spiritual dignity of vulnerable strangers—by its application of the Axial principle of caritas. Understood in this way, religion is inextricably linked with the goal of creating an enlightened, inclusive, and compassionate society. And as skilled actors charged with nurturing insiders and outsiders alike, helping professionals working in publicly funded organizations play a key role in defining that tie.

Scholarly interest in this care-centered understanding of public religion can be traced back to Max Weber, arguably the most influential social theorist of the modern era. Weber (1958a) first suggested that the process of rationalization—the replacement of traditions, values, and emotions as motivators for social behavior with concepts based on science and reason—threatened the religious principle of caritas ("love for all people") and could banish this ethic of caring for the stranger from modern public life. In some of his writings (Weber 1958c, 1978), he also suggested that if religious ethics such as caritas are to survive and be integrated into rationalized settings, they must become institutionalized through five key social mechanisms—authority, language, emotions, actions, and narrative. In separate chapters, then, I examine whether and how nurses at University Hospital assume authority and responsibility for patients' spiritual care, converse about spirituality among themselves, can experience their work as authentically spiritually significant, perceive and act on opportunities to address patients' spiritual needs, and use storytelling to manage the frictions between Western medicine and spirituality. Some of these mechanisms, such as nurses assuming responsibility for patients' spiritual well-being and performing acts of spiritual care, more directly capture the essence of caritas. However, they all contribute to the survival of this ethic in the sense that they add to the legitimacy and plausibility of the spiritual in secular care settings.

CHIEF TAKEAWAY

The main message of this book is that what makes religion socially powerful is caregiving. In the past, religion's power was largely a function of its ability to systematize otherwise irrational beliefs and experiences into doctrines and creeds. Today, I argue, religion's power increasingly depends on its person-giving and presence-enhancing capacity, or precisely what Weber felt was most valuable about the religious ethic of caritas.

Part of religion's humanizing function will still be carried out in the private realm by friends and family. But as the development of the human species continues to shift from small, informal groups like families to large, science-based institutions like hospitals, these organizations will be increasingly expected to provide humanizing cultures. That is, these facilities will not only offer the benefits of science, but will also be held responsible for offsetting science's impersonal effects by acknowledging and nurturing the qualities of clients that honor them as humans, including those of a spiritual nature.

Caritas cannot simply be built into highly rationalized institutions like hospitals, however. Nor do administrators tell staff how to implement spirituality. Modern organizations try to give themselves moral legitimacy by acknowledging the humanistic ideals of their larger society (Powell and DiMaggio 1991; Lawrence, Suddaby, and Leca 2010). But because these ideals conflict with these organizations' core logic of rationality, they are only loosely coupled to its everyday procedures. Loose coupling creates a "working space" within which workers can try to reconcile contradictions between an organization's rational procedures and demands and the society's broader and vaguer ideals such as honoring patients' spirituality.

Responsibility for balancing these competing demands typically falls to the workers who interact with clients the most. But because humanistic ideals like spirituality are at odds with modern organizations' principal logic, managers tend to provide few resources to help workers act on them. Hospital administrators, for example, give frontline staff little, if any, formal training in spiritual care (Balboni and Balboni 2018). This means that these workers are pretty much on their own in this respect: their organization provides support for meeting rationalistic goals like efficiency and accuracy, but when it comes to humanistic values like spirituality, workers must improvise.

Understood in this light, frontline helping professionals will play a pivotal role in deciding the fate of caritas. Specifically, to the extent that they assume responsibility for patients' spiritual care and talk among themselves about spirituality within their "working space," they will give caritas a foothold in society, a social and cultural foundation that will support individuals in their efforts to treat vulnerable strangers with caritas. Indeed, I contend that caritas is so fundamental to the definition of religion that if workers like nurses enable caritas to survive, that means that religion as a cultural and social phenomenon has survived, whether or not the people involved see their caregiving as religious.

I also argue that care workers' part in preserving caritas will be challenging and will require great commitment and dexterity. As I will show, a sizable number of nurses at University Hospital say they are willing to assume responsibility for providing the spiritual care normally expected of chaplains, but because they mistakenly perceive that their fellow nurses are uncomfortable discussing spirituality, the topic rarely comes up in their conversations. Many of the activities that convince nurses that their care has spiritual significance, such as tending to seriously ill patients, also put pressure on these workers to suppress their true feelings. Despite these communication and emotional difficulties, however, a significant minority of nurses are highly responsive to their patients' spiritual needs: as they work with patients, they selectively apply religious and nonreligious therapies to a variety of situations that cause spiritual stress. And most nurses keep the flame of caritas alive by crafting stories about their experiences with patients that suggest to them that spirituality and medical science are compatible.

The Meaning of the Terms *Caritas* and *Spirituality*

While roaming the corridors of University Hospital, I thought about how I should conceptualize caritas and spirituality. As I understand the term, *caritas* is not exactly the same thing as *care*. It involves more than sympathy or just helping meet someone's physical and emotional needs. Rather, caritas is only enacted when care has what I'm calling a spiritual dimension—that is, when care recipients are addressed as beings of inherent existential worth and caregiving helps meet their needs for meaning, purpose, and value in their life experiences. Moreover, caritas is a type of spiritually tinged care that is applied to all people, regardless of their religious orientation and whether they are an insider or outsider. As such, it is especially relevant to public life.

The meaning of *spirituality* is much contested, and the term is difficult to define; sociologist Courtney Bender (2010) has likened trying to define spirituality to trying to shovel snow. Nor did University Hospital offer much guidance. Like other publicly funded teaching hospitals, it intentionally defined spirituality in vague terms to make space for a variety of religious and nonreligious perspectives (Cadge 2013). For the purposes of this study, I understand spirituality to consist of all activities and beliefs that individuals use to relate their lives to some conception of a transcendent reality, be it religious or otherwise. Spiritual care, then, includes attempts to affirm and uphold that same transcendent quality in others, including strangers, so as to dignify their existence.[3] By transcendent quality, I mean the inherent meaningfulness and perhaps even eternal significance of every human being.[4] In suggesting that affirming this quality dignifies others, I am stressing the horizontal dimension of religion, which posits that the sacred can be found "here" or in "us" and must be actively protected and nurtured, as opposed to the vertical dimension, which posits that the sacred resides "out there," beyond finite reality, and can only be accessed through faith and mystical experiences (see Tillich 1945 for a discussion of this distinction). In this respect, my understanding of spiritual care is compatible with humanistic ones that emphasize faith in the goodness of humanity (Leget 2022). Within the context of this study, I also conceive of spiritual care as one facet of the holistic or person-centered care now being promoted by teaching hospitals. Hence, spiritual care can be provided in conjunction with other forms of care that address patients' physical, emotional, and social needs.

Having suggested how I approach terms like *spirituality*, I believe it is important to add what this book is not doing. It is not promoting spiritual therapies, suggesting that spirituality is a sure route to happiness, arguing for or against the existence of a supernatural reality, debating whether believers or atheists are more compassionate, or engaging in unproductive disputes about the religious versus secular sources of science. Rather, this book examines how frontline helping professionals' interactions with patients and colleagues make the spiritual dimensions of personhood self-evident against the modern backdrop of science, bureaucracy, and technology.

In that respect, this project is in keeping with Weber's interest in the plausibility and social construction of religion in modern society (Weber 1958c; see also Berger 1967). Later in this chapter, I will explore Weber's concern that rationalization threatens the credibility and application of caritas and how contemporary scholars have responded to and developed his ideas. To appreciate what is at stake in the conflict Weber identified, I first discuss how the clash between caritas and rationalization has evolved over time, the actors most caught in its crosshairs, and this conflict's relevance for modern society.

CONTEXT

A Brief History of the Conflict Between Caritas and Rationalization

People have long claimed that they are worthy of care because the group to which they belong has a special connection to the divine. In the earliest societies, certain plants or animals were believed to embody a supernatural force that animated and sustained the material world. Clans chose these venerated entities as emblems of their group's identity and etched images of them on stones or wooden objects and on their skin in the form of tattoos.

To be stamped by this virtual coat of arms not only signaled one's membership in a particular community but also set one apart as a sacred being whose fellow members were obliged to honor, safeguard, and care for. Conversely, to lack such a marker was to be considered profane and deserving of deception, exploitation, and cruelty. Indeed, as ancient societies grew into proximity to one another, tensions between them escalated, resulting in unprecedented conflict and violence.

But a pivotal moment in the spiritual development of humanity occurred during the Axial Age. Primitive religions were gradually succeeded by movements—Confucianism and Daoism in China, Hinduism and Buddhism in India, monotheism in Israel, and philosophical rationalism in Greece[5]—that extended the moral boundaries of communities to include those ordinarily treated as outsiders. Not all of these movements promoted a belief in the supernatural, but all of them recognized a transcendent element at the core of every human being that can only be encountered through acts of compassion. This ethos laid the foundation for today's world religions and spoke to the possibility of a new, universalistic understanding of care that effectively imprinted all humans, not just those in one's own group, with a hallowed insignia (Jaspers 1953; Bellah 1999; Armstrong 2006).

Adherents of these faith traditions have not always lived up to the ideal of universal care. Like their tribalistic forerunners, they have sometimes denied that enemies, unbelievers, and barbarians are sacred and greeted them with spears and arrows rather than open arms. But reformers within these religions have consistently denounced such parochial outlooks and argued that the dignity of every individual must be inviolable (see Joas 2013). The Hindu Treatise on Human Duty, the Buddha's "Hymn of Universal Love," the Jewish instruction to "love your neighbor as yourself," the Christian story of the

Good Samaritan, and passages from the Qur'an that emphasize respect for all human beings are examples of this cultural innovation.

These novel articulations of religion, combined with a growing scrutiny of magical understandings of nature, paved the way for more inclusive, effective spaces of healing in modern societies. Public teaching hospitals are a prime example. Consistent with the Axial Age's vision of altruistic universalism, these modern care facilities are designed to administer aid using impartial criteria to ensure that all people are given the same opportunity to have their health needs met. They also employ advanced equipment capable of manipulating natural phenomena and alleviating pain on a scale unimagined by ancient peoples, who believed that deities capriciously tormented hapless men and women.

Axial Age thinkers couldn't anticipate the constraints of modern times. In suggesting that caregiving would give intimations of the transcendent, they couldn't have predicted that care systems would evolve in ways that might threaten to undo the very idea that human beings are imbued with infinite value. Because public teaching hospitals render decisions based on objective, dispassionate criteria, for example, they can be indifferent to patients' deeper, subjective experiences. And by treating patients as mere biophysical objects, their advanced technologies may drown out ideas about the transcendent nature of the human being.

Caught Between Worldviews

That is not to suggest that modern care systems are soulless entities or that contemporary society doesn't appreciate its caregivers. But complaints about dehumanizing treatment are common enough that public teaching hospitals and other medical centers have taken notice. Many have sought to restore the image of individuals as sacred beings by promoting spirituality under the banner of holistic care. In U.S. culture, *spirituality* has come to be seen as a neutral and more authentic term than *religion*—one that applies to both believers and nonbelievers[6] and that invokes the idea of ultimate meanings without conflicting with scientific reason.[7] Today, nurses and other care workers are frequently recognized as "heroes" and even, as my nurse's button proclaimed, "angels." Especially during times of crisis, citizens applaud these laborers for their brave and selfless acts—though their status as "heroes" is often short-lived.[8]

Despite these efforts, spirituality's place in the public arena and especially in scientized care settings is controversial (e.g., Chopra and Mlodinow
2012). Proponents of spirituality argue that integrating this facet of holistic care into modern clinics provides a remedy to the objectification of
the sick and, especially when shorn of religious dogma, enables science
to develop in more humane directions. Critics, by contrast, dismiss any
suggestion that individuals possess a nonmaterial essence as an exercise
in speculative metaphysics.[9] They argue that assimilating such flights of
fantasy into care systems intellectually compromises science and furthers
human misery when, for example, patients' spirituals beliefs and preferences conflict with medical recommendations. Still others doubt that
the spiritual meanings that have traditionally undergirded religion can
be applied to strangers. According to Jonathan Haidt, "It would be nice
to believe that we humans were designed to love everyone uncondition-
ally. Nice, but rather unlikely from an evolutionary perspective. Parochial
love—love within groups—amplified by similarity, a sense of shared fate,
and the suppression of free riders, may be the best we can accomplish"
(2012, 284).

So far, these exchanges between talking heads have not included the
perspectives of those who directly provide care. This gap in attention has
its ancestry in the Axial Age, too: Axial Age thinkers did not consider the
views of their societies' primary care providers, most of whom were slaves,
servants, or women. Partly because the male luminaries of Axial thought
were so preoccupied with the aggressive behavior of their own sex, they
rarely gave women a passing thought (Armstrong 2006). In prescribing
spiritualized and universalized understandings of care as an antidote to
violence, these thinkers never consulted those who were then and are still
carrying out most of that supposedly edifying work.

Many of today's undervalued, frontline workers are expected not only
to implement the dictates of secular medicine but also to uphold patients'
spiritual dignity in the process. Are they able and willing to do so? How
do they understand the role of spirituality in their work lives? What makes
it easier or harder for them to uphold patients' spiritual dignity in the
sometimes-dehumanizing context of a bureaucratic, scientific hospital setting? Answers to these questions are largely unknown but are critical to our
understanding of the current status of the Axial Age value for spiritually
informed care of the stranger.

The Modern Relevance of the Axial Ethic

To appreciate the relevance of the Axial ethic for today and the role of front-line helping professionals in validating contemporary society's humanistic understandings and translating them into action, consider the COVID-19 pandemic and the moral challenges it created for essential employees in fields like health care. (By "humanistic understandings," I am referring to meanings that, whether couched in theistic or atheistic terms, acknowledge a transcendent quality of human beings that dignifies them.) In addition to dealing with the anxieties of infected people, many of whom believed that their lives were already discounted, these workers were required to enforce protocols that separated vulnerable populations from loved ones who affirmed their worth as persons. As one health administrator put it, "It's essentially like, we are going to keep you safe, even if it kills your spirit" (Englehart 2021). This requirement put pressure on paid care providers, who already felt overwhelmed by their technical responsibilities, to assume the fraught role of surrogates. This happened most obviously in hospitals and nursing homes, where COVID-19 patients were not allowed to receive visitors and care workers were the only people available to compensate for their absence.

But responsibility for care of the human spirit falls on frontline staff whenever we assign responsibility for at-risk groups—the young, the old, the poor, the sick—to public systems run by scientific authorities who demand that others respect their expertise and not interfere with their impersonal methods and procedures (Heimer and Staffen 1998). To counterbalance these organizations' cold nature, staff who directly interact with the public are frequently called upon to act as moral stand-ins and provide a "human touch." Teachers, for example, are officially responsible for imparting subject knowledge and skills that can be taught using monoculture textbooks and measured by standardized tests. But because this approach can easily damage students' self-worth, teachers are unofficially expected to praise students' efforts and incorporate antiracist activities to make up for this damage, much as a parent might patch up a child's wounds.

Indeed, the existential repair work expected of such workers has grown as responsibility for the development of our species has gradually shifted from families, neighborhoods, and churches to large, science-based institutions (see Perrow 1991). Ultimately, at stake in this rationalization of human needs is what, according to David Brooks (2019), makes us "radically equal"—the Axial notion that people are more than "brains and bodies," that "all people of all races have a piece of themselves that has no size, weight, color, shape, but which gives them infinite value and dignity." Marilynne Robinson (2012, 7) speaks of "a sacred mystery within every individual" and a "duty of creating social systems that honor . . . others with a type of reverence."

Some minimize this ineffable quality and the importance of safeguarding it in suggesting that today's social divisions can be healed simply by acknowledging that "we are all human." Just as conservatives' slogan that "all lives matter" downplays the reality that some groups are more marginalized and discriminated against, this argument overlooks the fact that there are competing definitions of what constitutes a human, some of which are more personal and compatible with a sense of dignity than others. Those who, like Peter Singer, subscribe to a philosophical anthropocentrism conceive of humans as having requisite traits like consciousness. Others, such as Richard Dawkins (2011), endorse a biological anthropocentrism, which says that humans possess a particular DNA sequence. In contrast, those who embrace a theological anthropocentrism, inspired by Judeo-Christian thought, portray humans as made in the image of God and possessing a soul. According to research conducted by sociologist John Evans (2016), Americans who favor the first two definitions are more likely than those aligned with the last to question the necessity of human rights, to say torture is allowable, and to believe it is permissible to end the life of a very old person who is a drain on resources (see also Camosy 2021).

As Evans also points out, most Americans do not endorse extreme versions of philosophical or biological anthropocentricism and retain a belief in equal treatment. Nonetheless, these two outlooks increasingly permeate everyday life, dulling sensitivity to matters of personhood. This is especially true within public institutions like hospitals and universities that specialize in complex problem solving. As neuroscientists point out, this higher level of thinking intensifies competition for access to neural and cognitive resources, causing mechanistic reasoning about physical objects to suppress social reasoning about the thoughts and feelings of others (see Christoff 2014). The mechanistic reasoning that is so valuable for problem solving is totally inadequate for understanding what people essentially are and what about them is of infinite value and worth preserving. It can also foster an insidious form of dehumanization that treats individuals as if they were machines (Haslam and Loughnan 2014).

Others acknowledge this impersonal quality of modern institutions but insist that it is a trade-off that individuals will simply have to live with if they are to reap the benefits of science (Serpa and Ferreira 2019). According to them, whatever insensitivity individuals might experience is only temporary and will dissipate once they resume their everyday activities. However, as neuroscientists like Kalina Christoff (2014) have shown, mechanical dehumanization can have far-reaching negative consequences for both victims and their service providers. It may cause "cognitive destructive" states, characterized by reduced clarity of thought, emotional numbing, mental inflexibility, and an absence of meaningful reflection. For example, as a result of being treated more like a number than as having a soul, frequently hospitalized patients may perceive they are worthless and a burden to others. Christoff suggests that these states are likely to become more commonplace as individuals grow reliant on scientific systems that perform everything from routine tasks to life-giving procedures. And far from being able to escape these systems' objectifying effects, those paid to care for others are regularly exposed to them. Hospital staff, for instance, often enter the health care professions because they empathize with human suffering. But because they must focus on the technical requirements of diagnosing conditions and administering treatments, they often must suppress their natural empathy. Without this empathetic connection, they can become alienated from the patient's sacred worth and from their own compassion and become plagued by feelings of doubt and cynicism.

MAX WEBER ON CARITAS, RATIONALIZATION, AND SCIENTIFIC VOCATIONS

The Spiritual Foundations of Our Shared Humanity

Max Weber, a close friend of Karl Jaspers and arguably the leading social theorist of the twentieth century, anticipated this problem. Weber was the first to note that in the eighth to fifth centuries BCE several important parallels in spirituality developed in the great world empires of present-day China, Greece, India, Iran, and Israel (Weber 1978, 441). But whereas others like Jaspers explored this era in detail (Jaspers 1953), Weber focused more on whether this period's universalistic moralities and egalitarian ethics could survive in the modern era. He frequently expressed his deep concern about the fate of what he variously termed "caritas," "brotherliness," "communism of love," and "world-denying ethic" (see Weber 1958d and especially 1958e; Weber 1958b).

This code, which different faith traditions have promoted if not always practiced, posits the sanctity of every suffering individual that others, irrespective of their group affiliations, are obliged to honor through acts of compassion (Bellah 1999; Symonds 2016). It abolishes the in-group and out-group morality characteristic of early human societies, replacing it with an understanding of care that is universal in scope (applies to all sufferers), personal in nature (requires face-to-face care), and acosmic in outlook (asserts that there is more to humans than their perceived physical forms) (Bellah 1999; Symonds 2016). In short, it infuses the afflicted with sacred value that compels others to care for and treat them with respect.

As he explains in the following quotation, Weber traces the origins of caritas[10] to the early attempts of salvation religions to deal with human suffering.

The principles that constituted the communal relations among the salvation prophecies was the suffering common to all believers. And this was the case whether the suffering actually existed or was a constant threat, whether it was external or internal. The more the imperatives among neighbors were raised, the more rational the conception of salvation became, and the more it was sublimated into an ethic of absolute ends. Externally, such commands rose to a communism of loving brethren; internally, they rose to the attitude of caritas, love for the sufferer per se, for one's neighbor, for man, and finally for the enemy. . . . The psychological tone as well as the rational, ethical interpretation of this inner attitude can vary widely. But its ethical demand has always lain in the direction of a universalist brotherhood, which goes beyond all barriers of societal associations, often including one's own faith. (Weber 1956d, 330)

According to Weber, then, the fact that unjustified suffering was not confined to members of their communities but affected all of humanity compelled salvation religions to develop a more universal ethic of loving and caring for fellow sufferers.

The Threat Posed by Rationalization and Its Paradoxical Effects

Weber feared that as rationalization in the form of bureaucracies and advanced technology permeated Western society, and as religious motives for action were gradually replaced by more scientific motives and understandings, rationalization would eventually extinguish human qualities like the spiritual that had previously ennobled vulnerable strangers, causing institutions to operate "without regard for persons" and dissipating the passion to ameliorate misery. This drive to rationalize human affairs would lead to a society that prioritized abstract modes of reflection like theorizing and calculation over the concrete, personal work of caregiving (Wilkinson and Kleinman 2016).

As the process of rationalization develops, Weber maintained, it also spawns other spheres that operate according to different values than religion: people pursue wealth and status in the economic sphere, power in the political sphere, knowledge in the intellectual sphere, an appreciation of form over content in the aesthetic sphere, and a sense of the natural in the erotic sphere. Weber feared that all these competing value systems would undermine caritas and relegate it to volunteerism and the private domain of intimate relations. He thought that caritas and religion would together be reduced to "ghosts of dead beliefs" and worried that modern people would all become "specialists without spirit" who, like Nietzsche's nihilistic "Last Man," would neither ponder questions of ultimate purpose nor pursue lives of dignity.[11]

At the same time, Weber thought that rationalization could cause unexpected harm to bodies, nature, and social relations. This harm, in turn, might periodically and paradoxically increase human interest in spirituality (Riesebrodt 2010) and stimulate an intense moral yearning to prevent future affliction and rehumanize relationships in ways consistent with the ethos of caritas. This change could be accomplished by positing that transcendent and sacred qualities reside within people that warrant reverence and nurturing. Religions, in fact, have long addressed the mortality of the human body, the lack of control over the natural environment, and the fragility of human relations based on differences in power and wealth. Weber thought, therefore, that the more people are exposed to crises they cannot manage using available scientific means, the more likely they are to turn back to religion and seek out new opportunities for self-awareness and invoke sacred understandings of humanity (Riesebrodt 2010). This reality puts pressure on care providers to supplement their otherwise mundane tasks with services that are of a more spiritual nature.

For this reason, Weber believed that caritas might still be relevant to public life. In his empirical studies of world religions (Weber 1958d), he held up caritas as a moral counterpoint to the increasing impersonality of Western modernity. Human misery, he pointed out, would continue to raise existential questions of life and death, and no other value sphere besides religion would be able to offer compelling answers to these questions. Caritas would thus remain as the ultimate ideal of virtue and a possible response to these existential questions (Symonds 2016).[12]

Indeed, Weber believed that as religions evolve, they eventually imbue the human individual with sacredness. Weber's suggestion that the sacred can possess and become immanent in humans resembles the ideas of an earlier scholar, Emile Durkheim (1951), who argued that modern societies divinize the self—that is, they make human beings ultimately sacred. But these two scholars saw this fact a little differently. Durkheim saw the social in divinity; religion, for him, was an abstract representation of the power of human solidarity. By contrast, Weber saw divinity in the social; religion, for him, defined the bonds and breadth of human solidarity. And whereas Durkheim thought that the sanctity of the self would grow stronger over time, Weber argued that belief in the sanctity of the self was inherently hard to maintain. From Weber's perspective, religion can never adequately explain why humans as sanctified beings should be subject to affliction, just as science can never fully realize its promise of a safe and painless existence. These twin dilemmas often come to the fore in care settings like hospitals where individuals struggle to make sense of their suffering and medical science may or may not provide a lasting cure.

Weber on Scientific Vocations

Weber espoused a similarly nuanced understanding of scientific vocations (Weber 1958e). He argued that science cannot provide us with normatively valid, universal truths. Indeed, it destabilizes the search for such principles by questioning long-held ideas about the importance of community, place, and self. For example, workers may gradually drop their religious identities in the process of being professionally trained due to an inherent conflict between science and faith or to institutional pressure to conform. And as the technologies that modern individuals increasingly depend on become more sophisticated, individuals actually know less and less how they operate, reinforcing the sense that their lives lack ultimate meaning. As Weber explained:

> What is the meaning of science as a vocation, now after all these former illusions, the way to true being, the way to true art, the way to true nature, the way to true god, the way to true happiness, have been dispelled? Tolstoi has given the simplest answer: . . . Science is meaningless because it gives no answer to . . . the only question important to us: What shall we do and how shall we live?
>
> Unless he is a physicist, one who rides on the streetcar has no idea of how the car happened to get into motion. And he does not need to know. He is satisfied that he may "count" on the behaviour of the streetcar . . . but he knows nothing about what it takes to produce such a car so that it can move. The savage knows incomparably more about his tools. . . . The increasing intellectualization and rationalization do not, therefore, indicate an increased and general knowledge of the conditions under which one lives. (Weber, 1958b, 139, 143)

Given the threat that rationalization posed to meaning, Weber was preoccupied with developing a particular type of science: one that would take as its main subject matter the question of what humankind's trajectory would and should be, particularly under modern capitalist and bureaucratic conditions (Hennis 2000a, 2000b). He writes that "the problems arising from the insertion of Man, a being capable of social action, in social constellations which in turn form these persons, develop their capacities or alternatively deform them up to and including the parcelization of the soul" (Weber 1978, 61). Because of his concern that modernity might sacrifice the spiritual dimension of personhood and thus rob individuals' lives of deeper purpose, Weber was keenly interested in such questions as the following: What are the origins of modern individuals' character structure? What are they becoming? What are the human qualities that the modern world selectively maximizes and rewards or, conversely, extinguishes? Does it facilitate or hinder "those characteristics which we think of as constituting the human greatness and nobility of our nature" (Weber 1980, 15)? In short, he wished to evaluate the sort of human beings that modern histori-cal circumstances were creating.

Although Weber thought that rationality posed considerable risk to human dignity, he didn't think the situation was hopeless. He held out the possibility that people could carve out spaces within a secularized world where they could still create and experience meanings. He suggested that scientists could rupture the seemingly impenetrable shell of rationalization by reflecting on what their findings say about the veracity of their value positions (Symonds 2016) in much the same way that students of poetry can experience a sonnet as personally meaningful by setting aside every-thing they've learned about the formal qualities of sonnets as an art form. Earlier social theorists, including Comte, Mill, and Marx, embraced teleo-logical notions of historical progress; that is, they saw history as inevitably marching toward various versions of a happy ending. Weber rejected this idea and gave much more weight to the choices we make along the way. Science, from his point of view, was always based on values in the sense that values guide what scientists decide is worthwhile and important to study. He wanted scientists to more carefully consider what values they wanted to support and decide on topics of study based on those carefully consid-ered values. From his perspective, these values must be allowed to shift and change as the complexity of life unfolds in its unpredictable ways. He thought that our choices of values and the way we act on them remain "per-petually in flux, ever subject to change in the dimly seen future of human culture, the vast, chaotic stream of events which flows away through time." He continued: "As soon as we attempt to reflect on the way in which life confronts us in immediate, concrete situations, it presents us with an infi-nite multiplicity of successively and co-existently emerging and disappear-ing events. . . . Life, with its irrationality and its store of possible meanings, is inexhaustible" (Weber 1949, 72).

In addition to questioning the idea that modern life will only get better and more understandable over time, Weber rejected a utilitarian under-standing of social science oriented to a "balance of pleasure" (Knapp 2016). He criticized political economists, for example, who focused exclusively on "the technical economic problem of the production of goods and the prob-lem of their distribution." Such an approach, according to Weber, imagines that "the only comprehensible purpose" social science could have would be to "devise recipes for universal happiness" (Weber 1980, 129). It would also fail to address the inevitability of suffering and the need to confer meaning upon it.

Weber himself tried to live out the ideal of a scientific vocation, but sometimes with tragic consequences. One of the striking features of Weber's seminal writings on rationalization and religion is that these topics were for him much more than intellectual puzzles. They were also rooted in his private and professional life (Wilkinson and Kleinman 2016; Watts and Houtman 2022). Weber suggests, for example, that his interest in the conflict between science and religion was sparked by the different outlooks of his parents (Mitzman 1970). He recalled Plato's allegory of the cave, in which a group of prisoners live chained in a cave facing the cave wall; their whole reality is the shadows they see on the wall, but there's a much bigger reality behind them. Likewise, Weber thought that his father's experience as a government worker had desensitized him to more profound kinds of understanding and led him to see people and their actions as mere shadows projected onto a curtain. In contrast, he thought that his more devout mother had a deeper understanding of events; she, he implied, stood on the other side of the curtain and was free to perceive reality in its greater fullness. Weber attributed his subsequent bouts of depression partly to his failed efforts to transmit the spiritual content of his mother's vision to his father's impersonal realm of science. Indeed, Weber described his professional life as a scholar as requiring him to endure the "antinomies of existence," suggesting that the pursuit of sociological knowledge exacts a toll on one's integrity and personhood to the extent that it reveals the painful limits of human knowledge and the value contradictions we all live out. In these ways, he personified the conflict that so interested him between caritas and modernity.

HOW CARITAS IS FARING IN MODERN SOCIETY

Scholars' Delayed Response to Weber's Concern
About the Fate of Caritas

Most of what has been written about the Axial Age has followed Jasper's lead and focused on the how and why its novel ideas took off and spread, when and where they originated, and why they didn't happen elsewhere. A fairly large body of work also opines about how the religious and philosophical principles of the Axial Age are worthy of emulation by government officials, corporate executives, and other leaders (e.g., Barnes 2009; Baskin and Bondarenko 2014; Tang 2016), detailing the accomplishments of a few extraordinary figures—such as Confucius, Plato, Buddha, Mani, and Zarathustra—who personify the various philosophical, religious, social, and political transformations associated with the period (e.g., Armstrong 2006). In contrast, scholars have been slow to address the issue raised by Weber about how caritas might survive in today's highly rationalized world.

One reason for this delay is that some researchers believe that Weber did not pay adequate attention to the "humanitarian revolution" of the eighteenth and nineteen centuries that fueled movements to end slavery, extend voting rights to women, abolish child labor, and improve working and housing conditions (Casanova 2012). In the eyes of many, this development infused humanity and care with sacred value and thus integrated the religious ethic that so interested Weber in modern society, albeit in more secular terms (Habermas 2010; Joas 2013). Rather than examining the impediments to incorporating caritas in public life, therefore, these scholars tended to focus on the motives behind its inclusion. There have been ongoing controversies, for example, over whether Western humanitarianism is inspired by a desire to alleviate human suffering or is more of a self-serving justification for intervening in peoples' lives (Seybolt 2008); whether the American health care system is driven by goodwill or is instead a fee-for-service model that incentivizes doctors to perform more intensive and well-paid procedures (Lockner and Walcker 2018); whether compassionate conservatism stems from altruistic impulses or the ambitions of the political right to dictate the lives of those receiving charity (Woodward 2002); and whether "aid trips" to places like Africa are actually about bettering lives there or are more about white Americans having the "experience of a lifetime" (Cole 2012).

Other scholars begin to approach Weber's concern about the fate of caritas in calling for a return to the biblical tradition of caring for others as an antidote to rising individualism and its possible (negative) repercussions. But when they turn their attention to individuals who are paid to care for others, they often focus more on their weakening ties to organized religion than the ways they might dignify vulnerable strangers at work. A prime example is the discussion of a young hospital nurse named Sheila Larson who was introduced to readers in Bellah et al.'s (1985) classic study *Habits of the Heart*, which examined Americans' commitment to traditional religious institutions and decried the increasing number of people who self-identify as "spiritual but not religious." According to these sociologists, Larson's unabashed rejection of religious authority and self-styled brand of spirituality—what she termed Sheilaism—smacks of self-absorption and is symptomatic of religion's dire decline (cf. Wilcox 2009). As put elsewhere by Bellah (1986), "Sheila Larson is a young nurse who has received a good deal of therapy and describes her faith as 'Sheilaism.' . . . The case of Sheila is not confined to people who haven't been to church in a long time. . . . Many people sitting in the pews of Protestant and even Catholic churches are Sheilaists who feel that religion is essentially a private matter . . . she [Sheila] has made the inner trip and hasn't come back out again."

Unfortunately, in mocking her individualistic outlook and blaming others like her for the loss of community, Bellah et al. (1985) did not consider the moral significance of Larson's work as a paid care provider. It did not occur to these authors that Larson, and other care workers like her who describe themselves as "spiritual but not religious," might play an important role in realizing their goal of reviving a religious ethic of compassion. Other scholars have gone to the other opposite extreme of ignoring helping professionals' spirituality altogether, suggesting that whatever spiritual inclinations they might have are irrelevant because they are hopelessly buried under a pile of scientific, financial, and administrative directives (Chambliss 1996). Neither group of scholars has investigated the place of spirituality in nurses' work—how they, as scientifically trained professionals, negotiate or translate such sacred meanings within a secular context and against a constant backdrop of human affliction. This despite the fact that nursing is consistently ranked by the public as the most ethical of all professions (Reinhart 2020).

Revisiting Weber

As a result of scholars' interests in topics like humanitarian movements and the decline of organized religion, there remained a gap between abstract, historically distant musings about the Axial Age and the concrete attempts of twenty-first-century frontline health care workers to enact caritas or provide spiritual care. Luckily, in recent years scholars have begun to fill this void. In light of the violent atrocities of the past century, attacks on the universality of human rights, the dismantling of democratic regimes, and the ongoing rationalization of social life, several scholars have revisited Weber's observations about caritas, suggesting that they have new relevance today (Bourdieu 2000; Boltanski 1999; Kleinman, Das, and Lock 1997; Scheper-Hughes 1992; Frank 2013; Wilkinson and Kleinman 2016). These scholars have called for a new approach to studying society that focuses on how people respond to social suffering and the meanings they attach to it (Wilkinson and Kleinman 2016). They also suggest that instead of studying affliction from a "professional distance," scholars must immerse themselves in local worlds of suffering to discover that it is in the giving of care that individuals are able to piece together a fuller knowledge of social life and its potential (Wilkinson and Kleinman 2016). And they recommend studying the moral dilemmas of caregiving such as the challenge of enacting substantive human values within highly rationalized systems.

They note that for Weber and other classical sociologists, the phenomenon and amelioration of human agony were central concerns. Emile Durkheim, the founder of sociology, wrote that "there is a host of pleasures open to us today that more simple natures knew nothing about. But, on the other hand, we are exposed to a host of sufferings spared them, and it is not at all certain that the balance is to our advantage. . . . If we are open to more pleasures, we are also open to more pain." (Durkheim 1997, 241–242). Contrary to the idea that poverty was the result of individual bad luck, Marx cited capitalism as the real culprit. He described this system as one that "makes an accumulation of misery a necessary condition, corresponding to the accumulation of wealth. Accumulation of wealth at one pole is, therefore, at the same time the accumulation of misery, the torment of labor, slavery, ignorance, brutalization, and moral degradation." (Marx 1867, 929). And Weber suggested that because rationalization seeks to organize human activity more efficiently by displacing religious customs, modernity struggles to create cultural spaces capable of both preventing anguish and reaffirming our humanity.

Scholars note further that since the classical period, the advent of television and the Internet has brought members of Western society into regular contact with extreme forms of death and destruction. In becoming "voyeurs" and "detached observers" of others' suffering (Boltanski 1999), Westerners have learned to distance themselves from misery, thus eroding their capacity for moral feeling. In the same way, the gradual professionalization of social inquiry and its institutionalization within the academy have undermined academics' original interest in ameliorative interventions and encouraged them to keep the reality of suffering at arm's length. In the words of Wilkinson and Kleinman (2016, ix), "Society was transformed from blood, guts, and anguish to an abstracted object of social inquiry."

Scholars suggest that perhaps nowhere is this tendency of thinkers to separate themselves from human agony and the ethical challenges of caregiving more striking than in Weber's own discipline of sociology. Although initially created with the aim of mitigating human suffering and being relevant to the intense moral yearnings it evokes, sociology has since been dominated by a value-neutral approach that keeps the study of the human condition at a professional distance (Wilkinson and Kleinman 2016). While this stance is partly understandable given the risk of identifying too closely with subjects and lapsing into sentimentalism, it fails to take up the original sociological question of how actors respond to suffering and what matters most to the afflicted as persons (Kleinman 2007).

In seeking to close these gaps and regain social sciences' human edge, these scholars draw special inspiration from Weber, who, as previously noted, conceived of suffering as a prod to moral and religious change, stressed how caregiving is torn between moral-religious understandings and the forces of rationalization, and advocated creating a place for caritas within science. Building on these insights, scholars have sought to address the lived experiences of victims and the meanings that "really matter" to them and have shown how rationalization—in the guise of state bureaucracies, mass media, and global capitalism—dehumanizes the anguished by denying their transcendent significance.

For example, to underscore the experience and meaning of suffering, Scheper-Hughes (1992) documents the horror of living in Brazilian favelas, where austere living conditions make children continually susceptible to starvation and distort the notion of "mother love" by forcing mothers to choose which of their offspring will survive. Describing his and others' experiences with diseases, Frank (2013) suggests that because suffering is a lived reality and not a concept, symbolic forms of communication, such as flowcharts, diagrams, and anatomical models, may help patients understand the chaos they are experiencing but can never capture completely what suffering is and means. And to reveal the dehumanizing effects of modern work, which is increasingly dictated by impersonal rules and technologies, scholars like Bourdieu (2000) report the suffering of teachers, social workers, white-collar clerks, and others who are denied a social dignity and struggle to adjust to rapid societal changes.

Consistent with the importance Weber attaches to care in vocational life, scholars who have revisited his work advocate for the actual doing of care as a means of learning about it (Wilkinson and Kleinman 2016). In this respect, they recommend a return to the type of social investigation exemplified by Jane Addams, who sought to expose the moral texture of social life through her care for a neighborhood on the Near West Side of Chicago (Addams and Messinger 1999). This approach differs from the public sociology championed by Burawoy (2005), which strives to catalyze discussion through the publication of books, opinion pieces, and other works and aligns itself with activists and various social causes. It also differs from professional sociology in that it eschews moral detachment and requires scholars to be transparent about how their own encounters with suffering might motivate and shape their analyses. An exemplar of this approach is Kleinman's (2020) deeply human and moving memoir *The Soul of Care*, which recounts the time he cared for his wife after she was diagnosed with early-onset Alzheimer's disease and describes the problem our society faces as the rising costs of health care reduce the importance of caring for patients (see also Frank 2017 on memoir as research).

Finally, in keeping with Weber's interest in caritas, these scholars go beyond merely documenting and analyzing what is wrong with the world. Instead, they seek to illuminate the moral challenges of caregivers and the obstacles they face in trying to hold social worlds together (see Tronto 1993). They suggest that, especially in the domain of health care, where care has acquired an almost entirely technical meaning, rationalization destabilizes individuals' sense of selfhood (Weber 1978). There, the rhetoric of risk, cost containment, probabilistic thinking, and mechanical information serves to "airbrush" the experience of anguish and reduce the afflicted to objects. To offset the excesses of rationalization, they argue that the dominant biomedical model of care must be adjusted to allow for moral-religious understandings that dignify the afflicted as persons and ideas about what it means to be human amidst danger and uncertainty (Kleinman 2007).

Scholars contend that whether these understandings and ideas are rendered plausible and rehumanize patients will largely depend on disciplines like nursing, medicine, and allied health that justify their status as healing professions based on their commitment to caregiving (Kleinman 2012). Other helping professions, like education and social work, that deal directly with vulnerable populations also play a critical role in affirming the personhood of strangers. As neoliberal policies financially starve public agencies, the challenge of reconciling competing rationalist and humanistic outlooks increasingly devolves to these frontline care workers (Hallett and Ventresca 2006).

Frontline workers also have a profound impact on how health care institutions are perceived, because the front line is where unexpected problems first appear and where those problems can be most immediately addressed (Lawrence and Suddaby 2006; ten Dam and Waardenburg 2020). As Felder and colleagues (2018, 101) observe, "Professionals do not merely create or maintain institutions. Rather, professionals give meaning to new institutional arrangements and governance principles in the context of their interpretation of other institutional arrangements already in place." The health care sector is currently dealing with just such an example of "new institutional arrangements" in the form of a paradigm shift from a medical model to a more patient-centered one. In that context, frontline professionals play a crucial role in blending established scientific priorities with new, humanistic ones like spirituality.

Remaining Issues

In documenting the dehumanizing experiences of victims, encouraging scholars to become personally involved in the giving and receiving of care, and drawing attention to the moral dilemmas facing helping professionals, this scholarship has raised awareness about the conflict between caritas and rationalization at the level where suffering is endured and care for ailing strangers is organized. A key issue that remains is how care workers respond to this conflict. In what ways, if any, do they turn humanistic concepts like spirituality into a reality?

In particular, scholars who have revisited Weber have yet to examine whether religious ideals like caritas might take hold in real-world setting through the five social mechanisms he identified (1958c, 1978). According to Weber, a value, religious or otherwise, can be said to be institutionalized in a local culture to the degree that its actors are willing to assume responsibility for that value, incorporate it in their day-to-day talk, relate to it emotionally, put it into practice, and regard it as believable in the tales they relate about their lived experiences. Examining whether frontline helping professionals transit caritas through these authoritative, linguistic, emotional, practical, and narrative channels, then, is critical to understanding whether this religious ethic can "stick" within modern care facilities like teaching hospitals.

THE CURRENT STUDY

Study Population

This book begins to address this issue by investigating the place of caritas in the work of bedside nurses. How, I ask, do these nurses incorporate spirituality into patient care in the highly scientized and rationalized context of an academic medical center? With the possible exceptions of medical social workers, home health aides, and occupational and physical therapists, nurses are the health care workers most immediately involved in treating the ill. However significant the medical diagnoses doled out by physicians, nurses are most often responsible for a patient's day-to-day experience while confined to a hospital (Rosenberg 1987).

Nursing, the largest care occupation, also has historical roots in religion but aspires to be recognized as a scientific profession and thus can be said to operate on the "edge of religion" (Bender et al. 2012). In modern hospital settings, chaplains are often viewed as the custodians and representatives of religions, and yet it is logically impossible for them to tend to every patient's spiritual needs, especially in the type of large academic medical center studied here. In fact, as other studies have shown (Cadge 2013), spirituality is ironically most present in these settings when chaplains are visibly absent and most absent when they are visibly present. This is because most of the images, symbols, and rituals that chaplains have relied on to legitimate their presence and signal to patients whom they should turn to for spiritual comfort have been removed from teaching hospitals. Consequently, when such needs arise, patients will frequently turn to the hospital staff closest at hand—bedside nurses. Because nurses address the realities of suffering and death that are at the core of religion and must justify their actions according to the logic of science, they provide an "acid test" of whether caritas is still possible within rationalized settings.

Academic medical centers are the quintessential rationalized institution, driven by the priorities of physicians, administrators, financial officers, and other experts and structured by an intimidating arsenal of tools and techniques that infuse care with a relentless impersonality. At the same time, because the United States lacks universal health care, they are the "last resort" for many of this country's poorest and sickest citizens. As publicly funded organizations, they represent what is left when society is disrobed and every private means of protection is stripped away. They are a symbol of the gap between society's aspirations and failings, where, "within the walls of a single building, high technology, bureaucracy, and professionalism are juxtaposed with the most fundamental and unchanging of human experiences—birth, death, pain" (Rosenberg 1987, i). To ease patients' anxieties and provide a more human touch, academic medical centers have recently taken several steps to incorporate spirituality into health care. The teaching hospital studied here, University Hospital, sponsored an international conference on spirituality and healing. It housed a leading integrative medicine program that regularly conducted seminars on the spiritual dimensions of care. In addition to hiring a full-time staff chaplain, the hospital created one of the largest clinical pastoral education programs in the Southwest; every year, this program trained four or five full-time chaplain residents and ten to twenty part-time chaplain interns. In short, the hospital made numerous efforts at the administrative level to legitimate spirituality's presence in medicine. This study examines whether and how these efforts filtered down to affect the actual delivery of medical care in the everyday work of bedside nurses.

Operationalizing Spirituality

As mentioned earlier, the concept of spirituality is notoriously difficult to define. I offered one definition that I developed over the course of my research and based on my interest in Weber's writings on caritas. My goal, however, is not to convince the reader that my definition is more theoretically valid than others but to determine whether spirituality is made manifest in nurses' work culture. In other words, how do we know when nurses incorporate spirituality in their work or render the spiritual plausible in their scientific setting?

To address this issue, I turn to Weber's writings on culture. As mentioned earlier, in addition to his more abstract writings on caritas, Weber elsewhere described several channels through which ideals can take hold in real-world settings—authority, language, emotions, practices, and stories. Building on these ideas, I look for certain signs that spirituality has been institutionalized through these mechanisms in nurses' work. That is, to answer the broad question of whether caritas has been integrated into their work culture, I ask how willing nurses are to provide spiritual care. Do they talk about spirituality among themselves? Can they describe their work as spiritual without feeling inauthentic? Have they recommended, offered, or provided services meant to enhance patients' spiritual well-being? And do their storied accounts of interactions with patients enable them to think that spirituality and science can coexist? To the extent that answers to these questions are in the affirmative, the Axial ethic of honoring vulnerable strangers as intrinsically valuable beings can be said to still occupy a place in modern care.

METHODS

Spirituality as an Organizational Phenomenon

To determine nurses' opinions about and experiences with spiritual care, a questionnaire was constructed and administered to a sample of University Hospital's nursing staff, the most in-depth survey on spirituality ever administered at a major nonsectarian organization.[13] Survey items were informed by presurvey interviews with nurses and other staff, including professors affiliated with the hospital's college of nursing, to ensure that the questionnaire was relevant to nurses' work situation. Survey participants were randomly selected to make certain that the opinions of nurses for or against spiritual care were not overrepresented. Having a representative sample of nurses also enabled me to statistically analyze predictions about the effectiveness of some of the mechanisms identified by Weber and to generalize the results to the entire nursing staff. Technical details about these analyses are in the appendices.

While there is no scholarly consensus about the proper definition of spirituality, nurses seem to have developed their own working definition of it. When asked in an open-ended survey question how they defined spirituality, 95 percent contrasted spirituality's inner, experiential nature with religion's external, institutionalized features. While not providing the analytical precision that academics might hope for, nurses' answers none-theless suggest that they have in mind the same basic phenomenon when answering survey questions about it.

Most studies of spirituality in nursing treat it either as an individual-level phenomenon (something embraced by individual nurses or patients) or as a property of dyads (something that characterizes a nurse-patient relationship). This study takes a different approach. I examine spirituality as an organizational phenomenon and ask how the hospital's nurses inte-grate spirituality into their work (Martin 1992). According to organizational scholars (Giacalone and Jurkiewicz 2003), an "innovation" like spirituality in health care will become an institutionalized part of an organization to the extent that the organization develops a set of shared ideas and practices that legitimize it. Studying spirituality as a feature of an organization's cul-ture is especially appropriate in the case of teaching hospitals because, until recently, they have tended to be indifferent or even hostile to spiritual care.

Indeed, academic medical centers are intimidating to many patients precisely because of their highly impersonal nature. As one administra-tor explained, "When people first come down here they sort of walk on eggshells because they have this vision of teaching hospitals as full of scary diagnostic procedures and a maze of floors and hallways . . . they are rushed in and rushed out, in and out. They feel treated like numbers." Adding to their cold character, academic centers have become increasingly cost con-scious. In the past, these hospitals were able to command higher payment rates both because of their market clout, based on prestige and consumer appeal, and because insurers were more willing to pay a premium to sup-port their missions. But that extra revenue is increasingly at risk as patients and insurers have become more price sensitive and less willing to pick up the tab for teaching hospitals' research and education. This change, in turn, has motivated teaching hospitals to develop a softer image by promoting spirituality as a feature of their new holistic approach to health care.

Combining the Analytical and Personal

Survey results and interviews are supplemented by accounts of two personal experiences. As explained in the preface, the first is about a six-month sab-batical I spent as a volunteer chaplain intern at the teaching hospital where the surveyed nurses worked. The second is about my time as a living liver transplant donor at a different teaching hospital. The chaplain narrative is written in the past tense and appears in italics in the following chapters; the donor story is written in the present tense and appears in boldface. By incorporating these two strands of material, I hope to pierce the veil of professionalism that troubled Weber and provide an example of how scholars can learn about social life through the giving and receiving of care (Wilkinson and Kleinman 2016).[14]

CONTRIBUTIONS

Advancing Three Literatures

This study not only speaks to whether helping professionals like nurses can enact caritas with rationalized settings, but also points toward a framework that is distinct from the two leading approaches to studying religion: the secularization (Chaves 1994) and lived religion perspectives (Ammerman 2006, 2013). Like the secularization approach, this framework addresses the scope of religious authority, only with nurses as its representatives rather than clerics, since in this context nurses have been assigned this authority by the hospitals they work for. How willing and able are nurses to act as surrogates of clergy? And like lived religion scholars, I examine the place of talk, emotions, practices, and stories in religious life, but instead of asking how these things help individuals construct a spiritual life for themselves and their group members, I ask whether and how they help nurses uphold the spiritual worth of vulnerable strangers. This new approach offers fresh insights into how nurses, as meaning makers and humanizing agents, instantiate spirituality into a job and a work setting that are based on a scientific logic that neglects this dimension of patients' selfhood.

This study expands on popular writings about the challenges and rewards of nursing (e.g., Brown 2016) by contributing to an emerging care perspective within the social sciences (Tronto 1993). In keeping with this literature's emphasis on the importance of integrating the ethic and practice of care in public life, it reveals the varied ways that a care facility's frontline coworkers can instantiate the same humanistic meaning of care and thus render it an institutional resource (Pagels 1989). By incorporating my own experiences as a giver and receiver of care, I also take a first step toward countering the type of social science whose reliance on "cosmologies and ontologies based on instrumental reason" obscures moral ideals (Taylor 1989, 74). Whether or not my accounts accomplish that goal, the hope is they will motivate readers to reflect on what Weber called the "antinomies of existence" in their own lives.

Finally, this book advances a growing academic interest in spirituality in secular institutions. This topic has garnered the attention of such disparate fields as philosophy (Taylor 2007; Solomon 2002), theology (du Toit 2006), history (Hanegraaff 1999), religious studies (Sullivan 2014), education (Wright 2000), social work (Cauda 1988), business (Giacalone and Jurkiewicz 2003), law (Snead 2020), medicine (Balboni and Balboni 2018), nursing (Burnum 2010; Ross 2006), anthropology (Asad 2003), ethnic studies (de la Torre and Zúñiga 2013), psychology (Pargament 1997), political science (Gill 2001), and sociology (Bender et al. 2013). Different strands of this scholarship theorize what spirituality is, prescribe its practice, and describe how people can pursue spirituality outside of religious institutions. This study shows how spirituality is socially constructed by a secular organization's frontline staff, who are charged with upholding the sanctity of strangers. In doing so, it illuminates how these workers can reconcile competing secular and sacred logics.[15]

As previously mentioned, Weber believed that if caritas is to survive, this religious ethic must be enacted in a way that makes spirituality plausible in public life. To understand what this statement means, it's helpful to trace the history of caritas up to the time of Weber and beyond and to consider contemporary scholars' developments and challenges to his ideas. This more recent work provides a better sense of exactly how hospital nurses might engage spirituality in the liminal spaces of their rationalized work environments.

CHAPTER OVERVIEW

Chapter 2 traces the historical development of caritas, from the time of ancient religions, when misfortune was viewed as retributive or deserved; to Egyptian and Mesopotamian religions, which understood health holistically as involving body, mind, and soul; to the rise of Greek medicine, which began to conceive of health care as a science as well as a craft; to the early Christian Church, which portrayed suffering as an opportunity to experience spiritual illumination by providing care to the sick; to the formation of almshouses and faith-based hospitals in Europe and United States; to the creation of public hospitals; and, finally, to a "spirituality in health care" movement within these organizations that reframes religion in terms of the more inclusive, meaning-making concept of spirituality. To give readers a preliminary sense of what this study's population is like, this chapter also presents survey results about nurses' spiritual or religious identities, their opinions about the promotion of spirituality in secular hospitals, and their views concerning the effects of spirituality on various health and social outcomes.

Against this background, the next five chapters focus on the five facets of culture that Weber's work suggests will determine whether the spiritually tinted compassion for strangers that exemplifies caritas survives in public life: authority, language, emotions, actions, and stories. Examining these factors is important because Weber's work was theoretical and stopped short of investigating whether these five media really do sustain caritas in rationalized and scientized settings such as hospitals.

Weber understood secularization not as the decline of religious beliefs, but as the shrinking scope of religious authority (Chaves 1994). He conceptualized rationalization as a process of differentiation: whereas in premodern times, politics, economics, religion, family, and other major social functions were all united, rationalization separated them into distinct spheres that each operated according to its own logic. As the religious sphere became differentiated from nonreligious spheres, he argued, people increasingly began to question clergy's ability to speak to these other dimensions of their lives. In the years since Weber was writing, however, some scholars have suggested that Weber's work overlooked the pervasive presence of the spiritual in group settings that are not usually considered "religious." In settings where religious professionals are absent, these scholars argue, "craft" versions of religious authority can still develop, whereby related professions like nursing learn on the job some of the knowledge and skills of clergy. And as secularized organizations become increasingly responsible for care activities that were once performed by churches, the jurisdictional boundaries surrounding the spiritual functions of care become blurred; in other words, the spiritual aspects of care are no longer considered to be the sole responsibility of organized religion, and instead spread out to anyone who provides care for others (see Abbott 1988). Chapter 3 investigates this potential expansion of responsibility for spiritual care by examining whether nurses felt obligated and qualified to assume responsibility for patients' spiritual well-being after their hospital announced it was terminating its chaplaincy program.

Weber pointed out that to create shared understandings, people need to share a common language: if we don't think that others are comfortable talking about a particular subject, we're unlikely to have conversations about it with them. Perhaps for this reason, recent studies of how culture is put to use in everyday life (Eliasoph and Lichterman 2003) find that people often work hard to avoid talking about the things that matter most to them, which ends up giving the false impression that they actually don't care about those things. This dynamic may come into play with spirituality: because it can feel so important, people may actively avoid talking about it if they think other people won't be comfortable with such talk. Because public teaching hospitals care for clients with a wide range of religious and nonreligious sensibilities, helping professionals are often warned to avoid divisive religious discourse and to use instead the more generic, inclusive language of spirituality. But even if these workers share an interest in spirituality and agree that it's relevant to their work, they may be reluctant to talk about it with one another if they misperceive their colleagues' interest in the subject. Chapter 4 explores this possibility by asking not only whether nurses think spirituality is important to their work, but also whether they think their colleagues find it important and how comfortable they are talking with their colleagues about the spiritual dimension of the care they give to patients.

Weber feared that rationalization would drain employment of meaning and human emotion. Today, organizational scholars find that when a workplace puts too much emphasis on efficiency and self-interest, workers can become so focused on those priorities that they become blind to the suffering of those around them and rob people of their humanity and dignity. Many of these scholars contend that this situation can be remedied by having managers promote compassion. Feminist researchers, however, warn that care is an undervalued activity susceptible to emotional exploitation, which itself creates suffering for care workers. So what happens when a hospital endorses spirituality as an aspect of care and asks nurses to care for their patients spiritually? Do nurses internalize their hospital's spiritual understandings and begin to see spiritual care as an important part of their work? Do they find that providing spiritual care makes their work feel more meaningful in a way that would help them keep doing it? Or do they find it emotionally draining in a way that makes it hard to keep doing it? Chapter 5 examines these questions by asking nurses whether they think of spiritual care as an important part of their work and what it feels like to provide this care.

Weber's writings suggest that the survival of caritas in public life depends on its being routinely put into action. His writings on the dehumanizing effects of rationalization, though, suggest that public care providers will increasingly have to choose between treating the afflicted as human beings and applying impersonal rules to them as objects. More optimistic organizational scholars point out that in everyday life, work is made up of small-scale, daily, situated practices and that care workers' ordinary practices may help them balance the conflicting demands of impersonal procedure and human compassion. Chapter 6 seeks to reconcile these conflicting perspectives by identifying why, when, and how nurses' spiritual care comes into play. The analysis begins with a set of common nursing practices that nursing scholars identify as spiritual; these range from prayer to guided imagery to the simple act of holding a patient's hand. It then looks for patterns in which of these practices are used by which types of nurses with which types of patients. For example, some nurses identify with their work roles more strongly than others, and some nurses go into that line of work specifically because they want to help other people. When these nurses provide spiritual care, they're affirming their own sense of themselves as deeply committed care workers, so they may find more opportunities to enact caritas. By understanding some of the conditions that are necessary for nurses to put caritas into action, we can better understand its chances for survival in public life.

When people are faced with the reality of suffering, they can come to yearn for a spiritual understanding of that suffering—and suffering is a part of daily life in hospitals. But, as Weber suggested, it can be especially hard to talk about these profound experiences in modern care settings, which are dominated by the language of science. One way that frontline professionals can reconcile the logic of spiritual care with the logic of science is by telling stories that put these two logics in meaningful relationship to each other. The more they're able to do this, Weber's theory suggests, the easier it will be for caritas to survive. Chapter 7 examines nurses as storytellers to find out how, in their narratives about their work, they do and do not construct spiritual meanings that are compatible with medical science.

Chapter 8 discusses what this study's findings reveal about the durability of the ethic of caritas in the modern era. It also sketches the contours of a new, caritas-based framework that complements the two dominant social scientific perspectives on religion today. On one hand, the secularization perspective suggests that rationalization has permanently disfigured the image of humans as sacred beings. The lived religion perspective, on the other hand, argues that the image of the sacred human being can be restored with the help of "spiritual tribes." A caritas-centered perspective, I argue, enables us to appreciate the pivotal role that frontline helping professionals play in nurturing and safeguarding that image in public life. It thus illumines an aspect of religion's place in public life that the other two do not. To demonstrate the usefulness of this alternative framework, this chapter spells out a series of questions for future research about the social significance of caritas, its place in less religious countries, and how it is expressed through other humanizing meanings and agents.

As a reminder to the reader, the text that follows consists of interweaving strands of personal and expository materials. Specifically, in each of the next six chapters, I will describe my experiences as a chaplain intern (in italics) that took place early in my academic career, followed by a systematic analysis of issues raised by those experiences (in regular type), and end with reflections on my time as a living transplant donor (in bold), which took place several years after interning as a chaplain and launching this research project. So, for example, in the next chapter, I first describe the circumstances that led to my decision to intern as a chaplain, then overview the history of caritas that I became interested in while working in that role, and finish with an account of the time my family learned that my dad needed a transplant. By so ordering these strands, I try to provide a sense of how the doing of care sparked my scholarly interest in particular issues and how those same issues continued to be relevant to me as the beneficiary of care long after I began analyzing them. Of course, one's understanding of issues rarely plays itself out in such a sequential fashion. Often one will, as I have here, revise and reframe interpretations after reflecting further on past experiences. Still, by splicing together these materials, I hope to suggest how my experiences as care provider and recipient motivated and colored this study.

Chapter Two

THE HISTORY OF CARITAS IN HEALTH CARE

What initially led me to consider volunteering as a chaplain was not a crisis of faith, a sense of obligation to serve others, or any type of supernatural vision. It was something far less profound: a need to get out of my head, coupled with a nagging sense that, as I had traveled down the pathway of an academic career, I had left something important behind. My yearning for "something more" was anticipated by Weber, whose writings warned that scientific progress and increasing intellectualization could lead to "disenchantment"—a loss of meaning and a sense of being haunted by the specter of vanishing religious ideals like caritas.

Seven years previously, on the day I had submitted the final version of my doctoral dissertation, I had sprinted three blocks to the northwest corner of campus and slipped into the Ohio State stadium. With raised fists and worn work boots struggling to grip the synthetic track, I had run a victory lap surrounded by an imagined crowd's deafening roar. Rounding the final turn and looking up at the bleachers with its thousands of scarlet and gray seats arranged in a double-decked horseshoe, I envisioned running a second lap if I were granted tenure at the University of Arizona, where I was to about to begin my academic career. But now that that day had arrived, the thought of a celebratory trot never crossed my mind. As I drove home that afternoon past Arizona's stadium and its drought-parched grounds, I felt relieved but strangely disappointed.

I had been warned that this might happen by a livestock breeder, of all people. During my second year at Arizona, we met at a university function for junior faculty members and their departments' promotion and tenure committee chairs. As the livestock breeder and I were both going through the continental breakfast line, choosing from an assortment of muffins, pastries, waffles, juices, and farm products, he introduced himself. He said that for the past ten years he had been a tenured professor with a joint position at the College of Agriculture and the university's Cooperative Extension agency. He added in a whisper that his area of expertise was the reproductive tracts of bovines.

Deciding to forego the beef breakfast burritos, I asked him what tenured life was like. "It beats the alternative," he quipped in a soft Texas drawl. "But to be honest, aside from the additional committee work they heap on, you pretty much end up drilling deeper into the hole you already dug. You study more and more about less and less." I brushed off his comment as I reached for some napkins. After all, I thought, why should I listen to a guy who makes a living researching the sex lives of cows? Of course, you would get bored if that were all you did. At least, I would hope you wouldn't find it too engrossing.

By the time I was tenured seven years later, though, I'd begun to understand the disillusionment he'd hinted at. My scientific training was not living up to its promise of "making a difference." I had been fortunate enough to publish in some of my discipline's best outlets, but that work seemed destined for the dust bin. Its subject matter—the dislocations and inequalities caused by economic restructuring—was also politically out of step with the times. As the country continued its neoliberal turn, the perspective I had been trained in—class analysis—was slowly falling out of favor in academia, and its place was being taken by a more benign, pluralist perspective that portrayed the world as a level playing field of competing group interests.

I was unwilling to jettison my interest in the harm caused by power imbalances, however. Indeed, I sharpened it by starting a new research project on the most potent corporate actors of all—fossil fuel companies—and the threat they pose to Earth's life support system. But like many other students of climate change, I was discouraged by the gnawing realization that the irreversible changes being done to our ecosystem were just that—irreversible. I would likely end up writing about a problem that had fewer and fewer chances of being fixed.

Adding to my unease was the endless posturing expected of me to build my reputation as a scholar. This was a first world problem, to be sure, but it was one I viewed with growing dread. I could not imagine continuing to loop the lobby and press the flesh at academic conferences. I had no doubt inherited this aversion from my dad, who would skip sessions at his ministerial conferences to take my brother and me to local pool halls. I still recall a plaque at the entrance of one that read, "Who is the happier man? He who has braved the storm of life and lived or he who stayed securely on shore and merely existed?" As a kid, this saying made little sense to me, but its suggestion that one might be unhappy on a safe shore began to resonate with me after earning tenure.

As my disillusionment with academia grew, I occasionally looked to my students for inspiration, hoping to recapture the idealism I felt I had lost, only to discover that it had been leeched from many of their lives as well. This was especially evident in their reactions to my obligatory lecture on Max Weber's thesis about the disenchantment of the world. I would begin by stating that, according to Weber, as societies modernize, they gradually replace superstitious practices with scientific tools to master and understand the natural world. Traditions and values are also pushed aside in favor of bureaucratic rules that harness and maximize individuals' productivity. I would then explain that these achievements came at a cost. For in demystifying the universe and treating subjects as objects, modern systems of control, calculation, and efficiency were draining people's lives of awe and ultimate meaning.

Before I had a chance to discuss with them what else Weber had said about this development, I would frequently be interrupted by a student—typically from the natural sciences—who felt compelled to defend this dark scenario. The student would argue that although technology is confining and bureaucracies are impersonal, it was necessary for science to keep religion at bay, or religion would ruin the advances societies have made. Other students—often business majors—would challenge the natural science student's outlook. Technology can enhance personal relationships, they would argue, and bureaucratic rules can be bent to accommodate human needs. Still others—usually from the humanities—would add that people can still transcend everyday reality through the power of metaphor and imagination.

I would sit back and let these factions go at it, sometimes to fill in the time but more often to mentally sift through their arguments, hoping to find in them a kernel of hope for myself. But they struck me as either confusing cynicism with knowledge, in the case of the first group, or as unwilling to face up to the reality of pain and disappointment, in the second and third. Nor did I help matters when I suggested that the iron cage of rationality that Weber described was slowly entrapping them. Their views only grew more extreme and desperate. It was here that a closet fundamentalist would sometimes speak up, arguing that such a human-induced fate denied God's omnipotence or something to that effect.

After spending years listening to such talk, working countless hours alone in my study, and poring over indicators of human suffering yet remaining insulated from it, I became convinced that some sort of essential energy was missing. I was feeling most intensely a failure to feel. I was experiencing what some might describe as despair but was probably closer to a deadening awareness that the thing I had devoted my career to had largely become an abstraction. I needed a break from what Weber called being a tiny cog in the great "process of intellectualization." I needed to spend some time where it was hopefully easier to shoehorn what really mattered into a naturalist worldview.

Sitting one day in my spartan office and staring out its grimy window at the university's medical complex in the distance, I began to reflect on my aborted plan of going into ordained ministry. Soon after receiving my bachelor's degree, I had attended a United Methodist seminary and served as a student pastor at a small rural church southeast of Columbus, Ohio. The town was best known for the foul odor emanating from a nearby paper mill, or what the townspeople affectionately referred to as the "smell of money."

I had stepped off that career path after my second semester, when I had taken a class in ethics that introduced me to the writings of liberation theologians who fused biblical themes of justice with modern work on class inequalities. I decided to deepen my understanding of social justice by enrolling in Ohio State's graduate program in sociology. My move was not without precedent—most of the founders of American sociology had been ministers or sons of ministers.

By now, though, I had not only trained and earned tenure as a sociologist, but also witnessed the slow death of the mainline denomination in which I was raised. Thirteen years after switching from ministry to sociology, it didn't make sense to make a complete switch from the secular back to the sacred. I still valued religion, but the thought of reentering a space that was slowly being hijacked by the religious right sickened me. So rather than choosing between the holy and mundane, I settled on a compromise—I would spend part of my upcoming sabbatical being trained as a chaplain at the university's teaching hospital.

Chaplaincy was something I initially thought would be easy, since I'd grown up watching my dad, in his role as a United Methodist pastor, visit parishioners at hospitals. But as the time of my chaplain training drew near, I began to anticipate the differences between the demands of chaplaincy and my seven years of studying society from the safe, professional distance of my university office. I realized I wasn't ready to take the plunge, so I tried to prepare myself by reading literature on religious responses to human affliction. I discovered that although the idea that suffering strangers are worthy of compassionate care originated with religion, religions haven't always looked so favorably upon the sick and poor. The hospitals that religious organizations helped found, meanwhile, no longer conceive of religion in narrow, doctrinal terms. Later, I stumbled upon books and articles about spirituality in nursing, which piqued my interest in what bedside nurses thought about the matter.

These readings helped to ready me on an intellectual level for what the work environment of a hospital might be like. At the same time, I still wasn't sure what it would be like at a gut level to work in such a place. As with many other people, hospitals had always struck me as cold and alienating. This tension between what I knew and intuited further fueled my curiosity about how the spiritual could possibly fit into an environment dictated by science.

I discovered when preparing myself for hospital chaplaincy that although scholarly literature on human suffering and religion could not address how someone like myself might experience performing the role of a chaplain at a teaching hospital, it did help me to put that type of work in its historical context and stoke my interest in how other hospital staff approached the issue of spirituality. In this chapter, I briefly review how religious conceptions of human affliction have changed over time, how religion inspired the creation of organizations committed to caring for vulnerable strangers, the tensions between religion and biomedicine within modern hospitals, and what we know and don't know about spiritual care in nursing. I conclude by presenting some findings about what nurses at University Hospital broadly think about spirituality, including their opinions about hospitals promoting spiritual care.

THE EVOLUTION OF RELIGIOUS UNDERSTANDINGS OF ILLNESS

Illness as Divine Retribution

As historian Gary Ferngren (2012) explains, in the ancient world, when knowledge about how the body functioned was scarce, there was little that could be done to restore physical health.[1] The causes of disease were mysterious and often attributed to vague numinous forces. When treating the symptoms of illnesses, and especially serious ones, healers would frequently appeal to supernatural beings for help using a variety of magico-religious devices ranging from amulets, occult objects like herbs and gems, to incantations and prayers. Diseases were classified and treated without medicine because there was no knowledge of medicine. Because everything that was not readily explicable was thought to happen for a purpose, sickness had meaning that could be ascertained by its interpreters. Breaking a taboo could occasion divine anger and bring about disease, but the gods could also strike capriciously.

The most common explanation for suffering in the ancient world was that misfortune was retributive. When the gods were displeased, they sent plague, drought, famine, flood, defeat in battle, or some other calamity, which could only be removed by sacrifice or purificatory rites that appeased the gods or spirits. A sick person was not viewed with pity but as a recipient of deserved punishment. Moralizing sickness by casting the ill as sinners in need of repentance was a late development in Egyptian and Mesopotamian religion, but it soon became common in antiquity.

Health in the earliest human societies was also understood holistically as involving body, mind, and soul. Mesopotamians and Egyptians thought health was present so long as life remained in harmony with the forces of nature. Similarly, Greeks viewed health (*hugieia*) in terms of an equilibrium or balancing of various elements, such as bodily fluids or matter taken from the body. Their best-known physiology was based on the balancing of what were considered four humours (blood, phlegm, yellow bile, and black bile). The Greek view of health also provided an analogy for the soul, in which moral virtue (*arete*) was thought to balance elements of the soul. This body-soul analogy was used by nearly all Greek philosophical schools and attributed illness to the failure to lead a balanced life of moderation and self-control (*sophrosune*).

An Ethic of Compassion

According to Ferngren (2012), in the fifth century BCE Greek medicine began to evolve from a craft into a science. Before then, folk healers had developed and passed on several unproven practices and thus failed to establish a body of theoretical knowledge, as is required of a science. Then Hippocratic physicians added theory to medicine and explained diseases in terms of natural causation. This more scientific approach existed in classical Greece side by side with religious ones in which the sick sought healing directly from a god through prayers and offerings, rather than a physician. Indeed, the best known of the Hippocratic collection, the so-called Hippocratic Oath, required those who took it to swear by Apollo, Asclepius, and other Greek gods and goddesses of healing to guard their life and art "in purity and holiness." (Many graduating medical students take a modified version of this oath today.)

Much has been written about the influence of Greek thought on the tradition of medical ethics,[2] how it formulated an ideal of competent practice that was subsequently adopted in late Roman antiquity and in the Middle Ages by Jewish, Christian, and Muslim physicians. Less has been said about how the Greeks, while not completely doing away with the idea of physical illness as divine retribution, nonetheless ushered in a new, more compassionate understanding of suffering that recognized the sanctity of all humans and gave rise to today's world religions.

In addition to conceiving of every individual as a unity of body and soul, the Greeks suggested how art, and in particular theatrical presentations of human tragedy, can sensitize people to the anguish and ultimate worth of others. As religion scholar Karen Armstrong (2010, 92) explains, for the Greeks, plays were "both a spiritual exercise and civic meditation, which put suffering onstage and compelled the audience to empathize with men and women struggling with impossible decisions and facing up to the disastrous consequences of their actions." As in the case of Aeschylus's *The Persians*, they pointed to how, even in the midst of a deadly war, shared suffering and pity can enable individuals to transcend hatred and see the sacred mystery of the enemy.

In a similar vein, Buddha, Mahavira, Confucius, Lao Tse, and the Hebrew prophets formulated a view of the human condition in which suffering assumed a positive role that it had previously lacked. They believed that, rather than bringing shame and disapproval, disease and sickness gave to the sufferer a favored status that invited sympathy and compassionate care. In their different ways, these Axial thinkers viewed misery as an opportunity for providing care for the sick and dying. Rabbinic Judaism, Christianity, and Islam were latter-day flowerings of the Axial Age. They rediscovered the Axial vision and translated it into an idiom that spoke to the circumstances of their time. Within Christianity, this compassionate ethic came to be referred to as caritas (Jackson 1999), which compelled believers to care for strangers by effectively infusing all humans with a spiritual essence through ideas such as the soul.

ORGANIZATIONAL EXPRESSIONS OF CARITAS

Earliest Hospitals

This philanthropic imperative to meet health needs is shared by all of the current world religions (Buddhism, Hinduism, Daoism, Judaism, Christianity, and Islam), although their organizational expression of it has varied across time and place. In the case of Christianity, which has had the greatest impact on care and spirituality in the West, early adherents of this faith tradition were enjoined to visit the sick and aid the poor. To facilitate the carrying out of this ethic, church leaders established congregational forms of assistance. Each congregation (ecclesia) maintained a clergy of presbyters (priests) and deacons who cooperated in the church's ministry of mercy. In the first two centuries of its existence, the Christian Church created the only organizations in the Roman world that systematically cared for its sick.

The earliest hospitals (*nosokomeia, xenodochia*) grew out of this long tradition of caring for the sick. These organizations were created specifically to provide care for the poor, the most famous being the Basileias, which was founded in 372 and employed regular live-in medical staff who aided the sick. (In contrast, the wealthy were typically treated at home.) After centuries of offering this type of care, faith groups in the eleventh century founded the hospice movement, which offered places of rest for the sick and dying as well as for travelers and pilgrims.

During the Middle Ages, ecclesiastical leaders tried to contain the outbreaks of plague throughout Europe by imposing quarantines. The clearing of these healing spaces apart from religious institutions had the ironic effect, according to Paul Slack (2012), of promoting what he called a "secular approach to epidemic disease." It was secular, not in being scientific, but in ignoring religion. This approach, then, began to raise questions about conventional theistic accounts that attributed suffering to sinful acts, suggesting instead that they may due to natural forces beyond individuals' control.

In this way, quarantines also prompted a rethinking about the proper place of religious convictions in public affairs.

Nonetheless, the fundamental premise of caritas that strangers are spiritual beings worthy of care continued to be influential and in the eighteenth century was a major impetus behind the creation of the first hospitals in the United States, many of which were faith based. Initially, these organizations were almshouses that provided shelter for the indigent and sick but no specialized medical care. Most retained denominational affiliations and sought to address the spiritual needs of the needy and suffering. This task was largely performed by nurses, the staff members most often at patients' bedsides, and retired or volunteer clergy thought to be incapable of dealing with the rigors of parish ministry (Cadge 2013).

Public Teaching Hospitals and the Poor

As historian Charles Rosenberg (1987) documents, out of this modest tradition of charity that sheltered and nurtured the chronically ill, deprived, and disabled grew public hospitals in the early nineteenth century committed to the "care of strangers." Rapid urbanization and economic expansion coupled with massive immigration and rapid strides in medicine also fueled the creation of physician-staffed hospitals, with specialized services and departments. As the middle and upper classes grew, many of these not-for-profit hospitals began reducing their traditional charitable role in favor of creating prestigious institutions that catered to wealthier clientele. Others, however, remained devoted to the mission of treating all people into the early twentieth century, despite mounting fiscal challenges.

During this same period, many urban public hospitals established ties with universities and medical schools to form today's teaching hospitals. These hospitals are uniquely important resources in the health care system. Besides providing numerous basic and specialized services for patients in their surrounding communities, academic medical centers are the primary sites for groundbreaking medical research and education. Teaching hospitals only constitute roughly 5 percent of all hospitals. However, they provide a disproportionate amount of care for especially vulnerable populations, including Medicare and Medicaid patients, hospital transfer patients with complex needs, trauma and burn victims, and those incapable of paying for medical services.

Teaching hospitals rely heavily on public funds to support their research and the many services they offer to the disadvantaged. The U.S. federal government is the largest contributor to research funding, which accounts for a substantial portion of the typical teaching hospital's revenue. Medicare also provides billions each year to graduate medical education. Because both Medicare and Medicaid subsidize a relatively large share of academic medical centers' patients, these "safety net" hospitals are vulnerable to any changes in these programs.

Like many of the hospitals that preceded them, teaching hospitals initially understood religious institutions in traditional terms as tightly bound organizations based on well-defined beliefs and recognized their representatives, chaplains, as authorities in spiritual care. As ideas from psychology and psychiatry about mental health grew more influential, clergy began losing the broad jurisdiction they held over the soul and personal problems. In response, clergy from mainline Protestant denominations began engaging these disciplines and established Clinical Pastoral Education (CPE) within hospitals. Following the institutionalization of CPE as a training program, CPE-trained Protestant chaplains began to organize as a distinct profession and established organizations to certify hospital chaplains, as sociologist Wendy Cadge reports (Cadge 2013). However, the smaller niche that chaplains created for themselves was soon challenged as well. Because it was still strongly tied to denominational outlooks, CPE struggled to address the growing ethnic and religious diversity of patients. Proponents of the biomedical model also challenged the value of religion and complained that it often got in the way of healing and curing diseases when, for example, believers refused to accept blood transfusions or animal-based products for medical use.

BIOMEDICINE

The Biomedical Approach to Health

The biomedical model is based on knowledge developed in the nineteenth century, particularly the anatomical and biological sciences. Its key practitioners are those with the greatest expertise in these areas. Doctors, for example, allocate resources, while other professions, like nursing and allied health, cooperate in addressing the priorities determined by physicians.

Under the biomedical model, sick individuals are assigned the role of the patient who is obliged to consult doctors' opinions and recommendations (Becker et al. 1976). When individuals become patients, their illness is also legitimated and they are given certain benefits (care, time off from work, reimbursement for at least some of the costs incurred).

The biomedical model excels at treating disease and delivering physiological solutions to conditions that previously resulted in disabilities or death. Its narrow focus on pathologies as the cause of illness and the instrumental relationships it encourages between patients and staff, however, are weaknesses. The biomedical approach works best for acute illness, when technical expertise is essential to resolving health conditions.[3] It works less well for chronic illness, disability, and mental health problems, when the challenge is not so much resolving a condition as learning how to live with it.

Biomedicine also casts doubt on the idea originated by the Greeks and later promoted by Saint Thomas Aquinas that a human being is a substantial unity of body and soul. Beginning with René Descartes, thinkers began to question this notion, positing instead that there is a split: that a body is responsive to the directives of a separate soul (Accad 2016). Scientists in the eighteenth and nineteenth centuries tried to solve the puzzle of what came to be called Cartesian dualism by identifying and isolating the vital principle that made a body alive. But when these efforts at grasping the essence of life proved futile or problematic, the inconvenient soul, which undergirded the Axial ethic of compassion, fell into neglect. Biomedicine, in turn, abandoned this concept altogether as a subject worthy of inquiry, reducing the human body to a complex machine that people hand over to physicians for repair (see also Frank 2013 on the colonization of the body).

Broadening the Biomedical Model

As psychologists Colleen McClain, Barry Rosenfeld, and William Breitbart (2003) note, despite these limitations, the horizons of the biomedical model have gradually widened to include the spiritual. In the 1970s, a biopsychosocial model of health was developed that drew attention to factors involved in clinical encounters, including patients' motives to seek medical care in the first place, their motives to comply with treatment, and the support they needed to change their behavior. Later a social model of health was advanced that addressed not only the health system and relations within it, but also other social institutions that influence the status of individuals, communities, and whole populations. According to this model, the goal of health care must be expanded to support individuals' capacity to participate as fully as possible in society, thus maintaining their identity as citizens. Most recently, holistic or ecological models have broadened health conversations still further to include wider cultural and environmental systems. From this perspective, health is the quest for humanness, and becoming one's self is increasingly difficult in a world beset by crises like climate change that threaten the basic resources (water, energy, food) needed for survival and well-being.

Each of these additions to the biomedical model has created greater space for spirituality within health care. Consistent with the biopsychological approach with its interest in the commitments people bring to clinical interactions, spirituality has been incorporated in medical discourse as a universal human need that must be attended to. In stressing how social support and participation foster health, the social model welcomes spiritualities, especially those of marginalized groups, to the extent that they contribute to this goal. And in shifting attention beyond the biological to the realm of human experience, the holistic or ecological approach recognizes that values, including spiritual ones, warrant being openly discussed because they will shape how vulnerable individuals cope with and are treated during crises.

NURSING AND SPIRITUAL CARE

The Religious Roots of Nursing

Although hospitals have broadened their understanding of sickness over time, the diagnosis of diseases is still prioritized, ensuring the dominance of physicians who are analytically positioned as holding the keys to this process. And yet, as Rosenberg (1987) notes, nurses continue to be the actors who most shape the day-to-day texture of hospital life. These care workers exert a normative influence that operates quietly outside traditional power structures but that critically shapes the "human element" in clinical practice (Fairman and D'Antonio 2008). One inconspicuous but important facet of nursing's humanizing role is its engagement of religious understandings of personhood.

Nursing, in fact, originated in religion (Bradshaw 1994; Burnum 2010; O'Brien 2010). As early as the sixth to fourth centuries BCE, the Greeks had goddesses who exemplified the aims of nursing. Aesculapius, the classical god of medicine, is linked to four female figures who have been associated with nursing: his wife Epione, the soothing one; and his three daughters: Hygeia, the goddess of health; Panacea, the goddess of healing; and Medtrina, the goddess of preservation. In the times of Roman dominance after the birth and life of Christ, many wealthy Roman women converted to Christianity and cared for the sick and funded many hospices. In medieval times, early nurses were often "fallen women" who took up care of the ill to redirect or redeem their lives. Widows who were left without resources were another group who often became nurses.

The association of nursing and religion carried on through the Christian monastic orders of the Middle Ages, the Beguines and Beghards in the thirteenth to sixteenth centuries, the Knights Hospitallers during the Crusades, and long-standing orders such as the Alexian Brotherhood that came into being when the plague (the Black Death) decimated much of Europe. As recently as 1900, church attendance and Bible reading were commonly required of nurses in the United States, and most schools of nursing had religious affiliations. And even up until the 1960s, it was considered customary and valid for nurses to read the Bible to patients, pray with them, and assist patients to "worship according to their faith" and "conform to their concept of right and wrong" (Henderson 1973).

Nonetheless, scholars have largely overlooked the religious roots of nursing. For example, studies of the founder of modern nursing, Florence Nightingale, have focused on those aspects of her vision that most closely align with biomedicine and her roles as founder, administrator, statistician, and theorist rather than her ideas about the spiritual foundations of nursing. Although Nightingale was no orthodox believer, she insisted that a trained nurse's capacities must ultimately be spiritual and that the appropriate use of the technical skills she acquired depended on this foundation. Because there was little physicians could do at the time to alter the course of a disease, she believed that it was nurses' duty to help patients attain the best possible recovery. She also preferred to train middle-class women, who, in her mind, were "women of refinement," tidier and highly efficient, and, in general, had higher ethical standards than other women. Hence, she endorsed a holistic approach that wedded piety and cleanliness and viewed every aspect of patients' external and inner environments as interacting to produce health or disease.

Nightingale's stress on the virtues of middle-class women proved to be a double-edged sword, however. While it helped to justify an autonomous female role in hospitals and created a dignified form of employment for women, in suggesting that middle-class women were uniquely suited for upholding the moral standards of hospitals, it implied that there was a hierarchy that subordinated nurses to doctors, who provided more technical expertise. And in using the "virtue script" (Gordon 2007) that women uniquely excelled in the area of values, the Nightingale movement cast doubt on women's ability to master new medical knowledge coming out of the natural sciences.

As a corrective, the movement subsequently sought to improve nursing's status by placing greater emphasis on obtaining scientific credentials. In the process, nursing's approach to spirituality was altered (Barnum 2010). Some nurses began to question beliefs in God and an afterlife as unsophisticated and products of childish wish fulfillment. Church attendance and scripture reading requirements for nurses were dropped as nursing schools gradually severed their ties with religious institutions. Course treatments of spirituality were reduced to reviews of the dietary rituals of major religions so that nurses might not tread on patients' belief systems. More generally, attributes associated with femininity, including being spiritually sensitive, came to be viewed as constraints on professional aspirations and not the basis of vocational legitimacy.

Spirituality in the Health Care Movement

With time, though, the excesses of a strictly technical approach to nursing also became apparent. Many observers complained that however illusory or superstitious patients' spirituality might be, the fact remained that in their minds it was quite real. Spiritual beliefs therefore might have physical and emotional consequences, and some ancient spiritual therapies seemed better suited to treat some ailments than scientific ones. Others, who favored a pragmatic approach to healing, argued that to dismiss spiritual therapies merely because they do not fit into existing medical theory is highly arbitrary. And still others challenged the idea that spiritual experiences are unreal, suggesting instead that they reflect the sophisticated workings of the mind and the complex nature of reality.

These and other concerns about the limits of scientific rationality led to calls for nursing to turn back to see what it had lost, to reintegrate spirituality into the discipline, and to make spirituality the "cornerstone of holistic care" (Clark et al. 1991; Nagai-Jacobsen and Burkhardt 1989). Several nursing scholars wrote, for instance, about how technology had desensitized nurses to patients' spiritual needs as well as their own, focusing their attention more on the functioning of equipment than on the interaction between subjects (Clark et al. 1991). Many argued that spirituality could no longer be considered only the responsibility of chaplains and that, of all medical staff, bedside nurses had perhaps the best opportunity to address patients' spiritual concerns about dying (Taylor and Ferszt 1990), especially those who work with the terminally ill in oncology units and hospice centers (Taylor, Highland, and Amenta 1999). Some wrote about the virtues of alternative therapies, such as therapeutic touch, channeling, and guided imagery, that seek to restore "spiritual balance" and how they could and should be incorporated into nursing (McGlone 1990). Partly in response to these New Age writings, religiously oriented nurses began importing their beliefs back into nursing and created specialty journals like the *Journal of Christian Nursing* that stressed the relevance of practices like prayer and being present with patients.

These developments, coupled with the fact that hospital stays were shortening, diseases were becoming more chronic, and treatments were becoming more technologically sophisticated, fueled a loosely organized "spirituality in health care" movement (Sulmasy 2007). Led primarily by nurses, this development framed religion in terms of the broader, meaning-making concept of spirituality. This shift was reflected in the Joint Commission, which sets policies for health care organizations and substituted the word *spirituality* for *religion* in its 1999 standards. While in the past chaplains had spoken of providing spiritual support, the meaning of the term *spiritual* changed from describing specific religious traditions to how people find meaning in their lives.

Within Western society, then, spiritual care of the suffering has been redefined as the locus of societal authority has shifted. Whereas religious communities originally provided spiritual care for their members and assigned chaplains to care for religious people only, today all patients are considered spiritual, and to varying degrees all hospital staff are responsible for patients' spiritual well-being. Hospitals have embraced this outcome as part of a new person-centered approach to care (as opposed to a disease-centered model) that honors each individual's dignity and understands spirituality as both a personal and interpersonal experience.

Today, spiritual care of patients or clients is expected of nurses (Ross 2006) and is reflected in nursing codes of ethics (e.g., ICN 2000), nurse education guidelines (UKCC 2000), and policy documents and nursing guidance (Department of Health 2003). For example, the International Council of Nurses (ICN) Code of Ethics states that the nurse is to "provide an environment in which the human rights, values, customs, and spiritual beliefs [of the client] are respected" (ICN 2000, 7).

This injunction is symptomatic of a growing naturalization of religion in modern society, according to legal and religion scholar Winnifred Fallers Sullivan (2014). Whereas it made sense in the past to draw a distinction between church and state on a doctrinal basis because there were established religious or legal authorities who defined insiders and outsiders, that has become less and less tenable as individuals claim the right to associate with or mix and match religious traditions. Beginning with the Supreme Court's decision in *Hein vs. FFRF* that religious establishment is no longer enough of a danger to allow taxpayers to challenge the government's promotion of religion, making the government "free to favor religion in general," public institutions are increasingly expected to promote religion as a nondivisive, universal aspect of individuals and imagine, therefore, every human as needing spiritual care. But while such care is mandatory in secular settings like the military (Sullivan 2014), where chaplains must perform religious rites, provide confidential counseling, and advise soldiers on moral matters, in others such as hospitals it is optional and thus subject to negotiation.

Nursing Scholarship on Spirituality: Topics and Debates

Partly because of its uncertain status in clinical settings, a disproportionate amount of the literature on the place of spirituality in secular settings (Bender and Taves 2012) has been penned by health care researchers (Cobb, Puchalski, and Rumbold 2012), and nursing scholars in particular.[4] The latter have addressed a wide range of topics, from defining spirituality vis-à-vis religion (Bradshaw 1997; Reinert and Koenig 2013; see also Pargament 1997), cultivating spiritual sensitivity (Catanzaro and McMullen 2001; Taylor et al. 1995), and improving religious literacy (Pentaris 2019; Taylor 2012), to assessing patients' spiritual needs (Taylor et al. 1995; McSherry and Ross 2002; Harrad et al. 2019; see also Pargament 1997), administering particular spiritual therapies (Taylor 2012), and testing their purported benefits (Matthews and Clark 1999; Lucchetti et al. 2019).

Most of this research supports reintegrating spirituality in nursing, stressing how its role can be strengthened by linking it, for example, with insights from quantum physics (da Silva Borges and dos Santos 2013), developmental research on transcendental consciousness (Watson 1988; Reed 1996), and other hard sciences. Some studies, however, argue that spirituality and holistic care are "fashionable nursing jargon" that make nurses feel special but devalue the profession's actual scientific basis (Gordon 2006). Others go further, suggesting that spirituality is purely a jurisdictional claim made by nurse academics to secure their profession's status that threatens to add to bedside nurses' already excessive workload (Paley 2006; see also Walter 1997).

The Missing Opinions and Experiences of Bedside Nurses

Very few studies of spirituality in nursing, though, have examined the opinions and experiences of its practitioners. Most of what has been written on the subject reflects the views of nursing scholars, giving the impression that the fate of spirituality in nursing will ultimately be decided in academic journals and not by nurses themselves.

What little research has been done on practicing nurses provides few insights into how they negotiate spirituality within their secularized settings. Many studies rely on convenience samples that are susceptible to selection bias and, therefore, over-represent nurses who have strong opinions about spirituality or are more inclined to participate in a study on the subject. Others are based on national surveys of nurses (e.g., McSherry and Jamieson 2011) or case studies of hospital units like oncology, where the demand for spiritual care is presumably high (e.g., Taylor et al. 1999), neither of which address how spirituality is variously engaged by a hospital's nursing staff. Adding to this problem are studies that only examine types of spiritual care performed outside hospitals, such as parish nursing (Solari-Twadell and Ziebarth 2020).

According to a widely cited review of these studies (Ross 2006), one consistent finding is that bedside nurses fail to agree on how spirituality is to be defined. This result is not surprising given that the term is intentionally construed broadly by its proponents. It does, though, suggest that spirituality is still being constructed and chiseled into a congenial shape at the level where it is to be applied. In addition, some studies find that spiritual care is rarely provided by nurses, or when it is, it is infrequent and unsystematic (Ross 2006; Narayanasamy 1999; McSherry 1998; Stranahan 2001). Advocates of spirituality in nursing claim that this finding partly explains why, according to many patient satisfaction surveys, the single most unmet need is care for one's spiritual and emotional distress (Williams et al. 2011).[5]

To the extent that spirituality enters the work of nurses, studies suggest that it only comes up when staff are coordinating care plans with hospital chaplains or discussing religious accommodations with patients, as required by the Joint Commission Mandate on Assessment of Spiritual Needs (see Taylor and Mamier 2005; cf. Narayanasamy and Owens 2001). Yet if Weber is correct that suffering brings spiritual concerns to the fore and that teaching hospitals are increasingly being held accountable for treating patients holistically as biological, psychological, social, and spiritual beings, there is reason to doubt such claims and ask whether they apply to entire nursing staffs. Extant research on spirituality in nursing, in fact, has yet to determine how spirituality is variously integrated into a teaching hospital's culture by conducting an in-depth examination of a representative sample of its bedside nurses.

In the chapters that follow, therefore, this study asks a set of questions based on the research on spirituality and the biomedical model in health care settings and in nursing in particular: Who do nurses at University Hospital think is best qualified or positioned to provide spiritual care? Are nurses able to talk about spirituality among themselves? Under what conditions do nurses think of their work in spiritual terms, and what impact do those conditions have on their emotional well-being? Do nurses who closely identify with their work provide spiritual care more often and consistently? And what experiences at work, if any, convince nurses that spirituality and medicine are compatible? Before turning to these questions, though, it is important to describe the nurses surveyed at University Hospital and what they generally think about spirituality in health care.

NURSES AT UNIVERSITY HOSPITAL AND THEIR OPINIONS ABOUT SPIRITUALITY IN HEALTH CARE

Demographics

Mirroring the characteristics of University Hospital's entire nursing staff, 91 percent of the surveyed nurses are women and 86 percent white, although younger nurses tend to be appreciably more diverse. On average, nurses have worked for 14.1 years in nursing and 7.5 years at the hospital. Their ages range from 22 to 64, with a mean of 42. The vast majority (93 percent) of respondents work 40 hours or less, and over two-thirds (68.2 percent) report that they are satisfied with their workload. In fact, the hospital was nationally recognized for being one of the few in the country to cap its nurse-to-patient ratio at 1:4. Readers need to keep this fact in mind when interpreting the results that follow because it suggests that one possible barrier to addressing patients' spiritual needs—nurses' workload—has largely been addressed in this environment, unlike in so many other cases (Gordon 2007).

Pro-Spirituality

Most of the surveyed nurses are broadly "pro-spirituality." As table 2.1 shows, 88 percent said that they are "personally interested in spirituality," and an even higher percentage (91 percent) considered themselves a

TABLE 2.1
Nurses' understandings of spirituality

Personal statement	Percent
I am personally interested in spirituality	88
I consider myself a spiritual person	91
I consider myself a religious person	42
All humans possess a spirit	96
All living things possess a spirit	78
Spirituality is a form of energy that can heal the body	86
Pain can be a source of spiritual insight	65
All objects are alive	19
Physical matter and spirituality are separate realities	54
The mind cannot exist apart from the brain	47

"spiritual person." In comparison, only 42 percent considered themselves a "religious person." This pattern is consistent with national surveys of Americans (Fetzer Institute 2020; "PEW Religious Landscape Study" 2017) that find a widespread interest in spirituality that is relatively untethered to organized religion. It also indicates that, like Sheila Larson, most nurses at University Hospital identify as "spiritual but not religious."

Conceptions of the Spiritual

As table 2.1 also reveals, the vast majority of nurses believed that humans (96 percent) and all living things (78 percent) possess a spirit, that spirituality is a form of energy that can heal the body (86 percent), and that pain can be a source of spiritual insight (65 percent). In contrast, there was a noticeable lack of consensus about dualistic conceptions of reality. Roughly half of nurses agreed that physical matter and spirituality are radically different things (54 percent) and that mind cannot exist apart from the brain (47 percent).

Opinions About University Hospital's Promotion of Spirituality

As mentioned previously, biomedicine originally embraced a radical form of dualism that dispensed with the spirit altogether and, like a colonizer, treated the diseased body as a geographic territory on which a foreign power—medicine—plants its flag and claims governing prerogatives (Frank 2013, 2017). Partly because of this history, the director of the chaplaincy program was cynical about his hospital's promotion of spiritual care. Researchers and administrators promoting spirituality, he said, "could be quite sincere . . . but they seem to be most interested in how prayer makes a difference biochemically, reduces tension, and helps to cut costs. That's not spiritual transformation. . . . They will still be skeptical that there is a divine reality behind it all."

As table 2.2 indicates, nurses have a more positive outlook. When asked about the type of spirituality promoted in secular hospitals like their own, very few nurses agreed that it is being advocated by individuals who are "out to make money" (7 percent), to convert others to their religion (4 percent), or to help workers cope with the possibility of being laid off (2 percent). Nor did most think that spirituality in health care is a passing

TABLE 2.2
Nurses' opinions about the place of spirituality in health care

Opinion	Percent
Most people who promote spirituality in hospitals are out to make money	7
People who promote spirituality in hospitals are trying to convert others to their religion	4
The real reason spirituality is being promoted in hospitals is to help workers cope with the possibility of being laid off	2
Spirituality is a fad	8
Spirituality is becoming too commercialized	30
The kind of spirituality being promoted in hospitals is superficial	26
Spirituality is being promoted in hospitals because patients' spiritual needs have been neglected in the past	70
Hospitals should be concerned about the spirituality of their nurses	72
Promoting spirituality in hospitals may diminish the importance of organized religion	3
Promoting spirituality in hospitals is at odds with the real purpose of medicine	4
Science and technology can discourage a belief in spiritual matters	51

"fad" (8 percent), is becoming too commercialized (30 percent), and is superficial in nature (26 percent). Rather, a majority (70 percent) felt that spirituality is now being promoted because patients' spiritual needs had been neglected in the past.

This last point was echoed by nurses and others in presurvey interviews. A nurse in the cardiology unit applauded the hospital for being more "culturally sensitive" and "accepting all people," especially its efforts to "accommodate the preferences of our Native American population." Similarly, the head of Nursing Services stressed that "we teach the staff to respect cultural diversity and to ask patients, what is important to you? . . . Rather than just make generalized assumptions like 'Oh, they're Native American, so we should get a medicine man to come see them.'" A trained nurse and head of Adult Services explained that, in promoting spirituality, "We're sort of swinging back in terms of looking at all aspects of a person . . . it hasn't emanated from nursing per se, but it's come from outside sources."

Along the same lines, a member of the hospital's integrative medicine program explained, "I don't think it is a fad. It's kind of an appreciation of a missing element in people's lives." A doctor from Family and Community Medicine believed that the hospital's interest in spirituality stemmed from "the alienation brought on by technological culture . . . the realization that that's not what creates the meaning and purpose of life . . . it is a cultural and social movement." A physician who works with chronically ill children added that "people are giving us permission to make spirituality a part of their care."

As table 2.2 also shows, far from thinking that hospitals are being intrusive in advocating spirituality and that it should be treated as a private matter, most surveyed nurses agreed that hospitals should be concerned about the spirituality of their nurses (72 percent). And virtually none believed that promoting spirituality diminishes the importance of religion (3 percent) or is at odds with the real purpose of medicine (4 percent). At the same time, a little over half of them agreed that science and technology can discourage a belief in spiritual matters (51 percent). A few of the interviewed nurses also felt that popular culture promoted understandings of spirituality that they, as highly trained professionals, found to be childish and, in some respects, demeaning. As one nurse who took spirituality quite seriously explained, "I am irritated by all these cutesy pictures of angels and stuff like that . . . There is this whole spiritual system created out of them. It doesn't really explain things to me appropriately. I recognize that there are very strong spiritual forces out there. . . . But when I see things like, you know, pictures of cute little babies with wings, I am offended by it."

The Efficacy and Inclusivity of Spirituality

Nurses were asked whether they believed that spirituality could produce certain effects in patients (see table 2.3). The vast majority felt that spirituality could give their patients inner peace (100 percent), give them strength to cope (98 percent), bring about physical relaxation (97 percent) and self-awareness (96 percent), and help them to forgive (93 percent), connect (94 percent), and cooperate with others (92 percent). Between 75 and 90 percent believed that spirituality could reduce bodily pain (85 percent), provide an experience of God's forgiveness (83 percent), give assurances of eternal life (78 percent), produce physical healing through the powers of the mind (78 percent), and help patients discover the deeper meaning of their illness (77 percent). A slightly smaller percentage (61–70 percent) of the nurses thought that spirituality could facilitate physical healing by God or some cosmic force (70 percent), assist in the discovery of the deeper meaning of one's pain (68 percent), and produce an altered state of consciousness

TABLE 2.3
Nurses' beliefs about the effects of spirituality in patients

Effect	Percent
Inner peace	100
Strength to cope	98
Physical relaxation	97
Self-awareness	96
A greater sense of connection with others	94
Forgiveness of others	93
A more cooperative attitude	92
Reduction in physical pain	85
An experience of God's forgiveness	83
Physical healing through the powers of the mind	78
Assurance of eternal life	78
Discovery of the deeper meaning of one's illness	77
Physical healing by God or some cosmic force	70
Discovery of the deeper meaning of one's pain	68
An altered state of consciousness, e.g., mystic state	61
Financial success	35
A nurse's spirituality can improve the quality of care patients receive	84
Nurses should pray for patients when asked, even if they do not feel qualified to do so	34

(61 percent). Of the questions asked, financial success was the only effect most nurses did not think spirituality could create for patients (35 percent).

Interestingly, nurses felt that their own spirituality had consequences, but some expressed reservations about being required to provide spiritual care of a religious nature. Well over three-fourths (84 percent) of nurses agreed that a nurse's spirituality can improve the quality of care that patients receive. But only about a third (34 percent) of respondents thought that nurses should pray for patients when asked, even if they do not feel qualified to do so.

It was especially noteworthy that, unlike religious and secular fundamentalists, who use divisive and uncompromising rhetoric, nurses tend to discuss spirituality in inclusive and pragmatic terms. One interviewed nurse, for example, said that he tried "to be more accepting of other people's spirituality, no matter where they come from, whether they are Native

American, Baptist, or Jew. I can take some of what they're saying and integrate it into the context of my belief system. It doesn't go against anything that I believe in. I find it very peaceful." He concluded, "So, I just give them something in return to build on. Something that's within their own belief." A professor in the Nursing College echoed this pragmatic approach when she said that "for me the importance of spirituality is as a resource. As a nurse, my goal would be to see how it can enhance overall well-being . . . So, it's more an independent variable."

In general, nurses view their hospital's promotion of spirituality as an acknowledgment that people are humans, not machines, and they conceive of the spiritual as a dimension of being human that suffering accentuates. Spirituality can also make care work like nursing morally intense and significant. In the words of one nurse, "To me, spirituality is about living your life every single day with integrity, being open to seeing the beauty in every person." Commenting on the inescapable presence of suffering in hospitals, another nurse of twenty-five years stated, "It's still exciting to see a baby born after all of these years. It can be fun. But it can also be the saddest place on earth . . . being a nurse has definitely got to be the most stressful but the most rewarding job at the same time." In the chapters that follow, we will explore whether administrators' promotion of spirituality and nurses' positive attitudes about it result in a widespread integration of spirituality into nurses' care of the afflicted.

While spirituality is something broadly supported by the hospital but left to the discretion of nurses, this is much less likely to be true of their patients. For many patients, the experience of affliction can make ultimate concerns like the spiritual inescapable. Any spiritual angst they may feel is then exacerbated by our health care system, which often treats patients as sick bodies to be reconfigured by bureaucracies run by experts. The sick person and their loved ones may find themselves in the desperate position of having to navigate these highly complex and impersonal systems during a time of considerable stress. This was my experience when my family and I sought out a liver transplant for my dad.

Several years after I trained as a chaplain intern at a hospital, my family and I are now knocking on the doors of other medical facilities, this time hoping to find one willing to admit my dad and perform a living donor liver transplant. The first surgeon we meet with runs a clinic near

my parents' condo in Phoenix. Before driving there, our entire family—
my dad, mom, brother, sister, and myself—gather at my parents' home.
Sitting together in their poorly insulated patio room, none of us knowing whether we should get our hopes up, I recall the events leading to
this moment.

Nearly ten years ago, on the day after my sister's wedding, my mom
noticed that my dad's eyes seemed jaundiced. He went to be tested, and
the initial results suggested he might have liver cancer. However, it was
later determined that he had primary sclerosing cholangitis, a disease
that causes scarring of the liver's bile ducts, which is an equally fatal
condition. He was treated with a drug called Actigall, which slowed the
disease's progression. But the medication slowly began to lose its effectiveness after three years. Fatigue set in, the abdominal pain intensified,
and his eyes and skin more regularly became a sickly yellow. My dad's
mental functions were also increasingly compromised by the ammonia
seeping from the liver to the brain.

Because my dad is a nonsmoker and still manages to walk five miles
three times a week, he is in theory a good candidate for a transplant.
Yet because he is seventy and considered a greater statistical risk, he is
so far down the waiting list that it is highly unlikely that he will survive
long enough to receive a cadaver's liver. Our family scours the Internet for options that would not require such a lengthy wait. We eventually learn of an alternative to deceased donor organ transplantation—a
living donor liver transplant procedure. With this procedure, surgeons
remove a 40–60 percent segment of a living donor's healthy liver. They
then remove the recipient's entire diseased liver and replace it with the
donor's excised portion. Both the donor's and recipient's liver grow back
to their full size within weeks, proving, I suppose, that tales of Pro-
metheus's regenerative liver were not so far-fetched after all. The major
challenge of this controversial procedure is not just finding a willing
donor, but one whose liver size, blood, and tissue type match those of
the recipient. In my dad's case, we face the additional obstacle of finding a transplant center willing to operate on an older, high-risk patient.

The organ transplant center at the University of Pittsburgh Medical Center (UPMC) is the largest in the world, performing a deceased
donor operation every day and the more controversial, living donor version nearly once every two weeks. Because of its size and international

reputation, UPMC can afford to take greater risks than most other centers. We are excited to speak with the surgeon at the clinic near my parents' house after learning he was trained at the UPMC's organ transplant center.

Around noon we get in my brother's car and drive to the clinic. We review the questions we want to ask the surgeon, punctuating our discussion with long, awkward stretches of silence. It is the middle of July, and a heat mirage floats over the clinic's blacktop parking lot as we pull in. Getting out of the car, we squint when assailed by the sun's intense glare and reflections off the side mirrors and hubcaps of the vehicles parked around us. We quietly make our way to the clinic's entry, where we walk under a canopy's cooler shadows and then are blasted with the chill of air conditioning on the other side of a glass door.

We sit in the waiting room for over an hour, occasionally glancing at but never opening old issues of *Time*, *Woman's Day*, and *Arizona Highways* set on a table. When the surgeon finally comes out, he leads us back to his office. He reminds me of a well-to-do orthodontist who fitted my braces as a teen and whom I never fully trusted—a silver-haired, bronze-faced man in his late sixties with unnaturally warm and clean hands. Before we have a chance to pose our questions, the surgeon discusses in dizzying detail the results of an MRI taken three days earlier.

He concludes his exhausting assessment by bringing up a scan on his computer and pointing out that my dad has a "clogged portal vein." He explains that "the etiology is not fully understood, but it is based on thrombotic tendency related to several factors: altered liver anatomy that increases the intrahepatic resistance to portal flow, endothelial injury due to an elevated portal pressure, and coagulation abnormalities. It is considered a contraindication for liver transplantation but the clinic is happy to admit your dad and take care of him."

He smiles so widely and abruptly when he finishes that we feel that we have been congratulated. Later, as we trudge through the heat back to the car, no one speaks until my brother comments, "Well, the surgeon seemed hopeful."

"But wasn't he saying that dad's condition prevented him from having a transplant?" my sister gravely asks.

It is not until we get into the car and finish processing what exactly the surgeon said that we understand that the prognosis is dire and the surgeon was merely offering our dad palliative care for his last days.

We had assumed that the surgeon was in regular contact with UPMC and therefore familiar with the most recent developments in living donor transplantation. It turns out that he is not. By chance, we discover later that day on the Internet that while it was once true that a clogged portal valve precluded a living donor transplantation, that is no longer the case because UPMC has recently devised a technique that circumvents this problem. And yet the surgeon acted like he knew everything there was to know about transplants.

The next morning, we contact UPMC directly to see if they will consider our dad as a patient. A nurse who coordinates the transplant procedure says the hospital will work with Dad, provided we find some potential living donors and both the donors and Dad are willing to undergo a series of rigorous evaluation tests to determine whether they are a good match. All three siblings are willing to serve as donors and have their respective families' blessing to do so. Because my build—and presumably my liver—are closest in size to my dad's, it is decided that I will be evaluated first.

We buy tickets to fly Dad and me from Phoenix to Pittsburgh that night. So much ammonia is now traveling from Dad's diseased liver to his brain that he is often confused and blurts out inappropriate comments. As we sit next to each other on the plane, I do my best to calm him and contain his remarks. He grows anxious when the attendants are slow to collect his empty plastic cup and cookie wrapper and blurts to a woman across the aisle that there must be something wrong that the crew is not telling us about. I distract him by drawing his attention to the moonlit clouds seen through the window to his left. He stares intensely for minutes at a time at the glowing, billowing masses, as if trying to discern something that lies beyond them, until his eyes, reflected in the porthole, slowly begin to water from the strain.

As I watch him grow anxious, I think about the conversation with the nurse at UPMC. She is the only one at the hospital we have spoken with so far about the possibility of a liver transplant. It strikes me that very soon care for Dad's ailing body and spirit could be transferred entirely out of my family's hands into those of workers like herself. To them, he is a complete stranger. Could they possibly value him in the same way that we do?

Chapter Three

CRAFT VERSIONS OF RELIGIOUS AUTHORITY

Who is qualified to give strangers spiritual care in today's highly scientized settings? I began to ask myself this question while I was traveling to the university hospital and wondering whether I would be accepted into its chaplaincy program. Were they looking for someone familiar with the customs, habits, and routines of the church? I was, but I was uncomfortable with many of the expectations placed on clergy, such as wearing a clerical collar and referring to oneself as Reverend. Were they wishing for someone with expertise in running religious governments and enforcing its laws? I had no such experience, nor was I wanting to acquire it. Were they wanting someone who was a visionary and possessed special "spiritual gifts"? That was not the case with me either. None of these traditional, legal, and charismatic understandings of authority, which Weber suggested were critical to the survival of religion, seemed to apply to me. Indeed, it was unclear to me on what authority anyone could give spiritual care in an academic medical center. And yet if Weber was correct, the fate of caritas hinged on some type of individual assuming responsibility for it.

After arriving at the hospital, I spent nearly thirty minutes combing its halls trying to find the office of the director of the Clinical Pastoral Education (CPE) program, who was to interview me for a chaplain intern position. As I anxiously waited for an elevator to descend four floors to my level, my sense of inadequacy grew and I felt less and less fit for the role. When I finally found the office in a remote corner on the second floor, I knocked but no one answered. Thinking a waiting room must be on the other side, I walked in and was startled to discover that the room led directly into the office of the director, who was seated erectly behind an executive desk wearing headphones and a double-breasted suit.

His desktop was dominated by a framed picture of a woman who I presumed was his wife but later learned was his guru. He seemed agitated by my abrupt entrance but removed his headphones and rose to shake my hand and offer me a chair. Thumbing through the written application that I had mailed him a month earlier, he asked me to elaborate on the summary of my spiritual background, which I had kept deliberately brief because I did not feel comfortable confiding in someone like himself whom I had never met. He then asked if I had any past experiences that might interfere with my ability to work in a hospital setting and relate to patients as a chaplain. He also inquired about my future career goals. I explained that I could not think of anything that would compromise my performance as chaplain and my career goals were, at the moment, undecided. As he rapidly tapped his fingers, I grew awkward, sensing that I was not giving him the answers he needed or hoped for. He sighed, exhaled, and then, to my surprise, informed me that I had been accepted. He instructed me to go the next morning to two tan mobile units behind the hospital to fill out medical forms and get security clearance.

I arrived at the units at 9:00 A.M. just as they were opening for business. The first unit was run by a traveling nurse from Pakistan. Its reception area, where I signed the forms, was covered with simulated wood paneling; two large posters hung on the wall behind the counter. The first quoted a British theologian I had never heard of about how change, whether for good or not, is always difficult. The second listed and scored various snack items for their nutritional value. Kale chips were at the top. I suspected the two posters were meant to speak to the value of holistic care or something along those lines, but I could not help but be struck by their awkward juxtaposition of the spiritual and material.

The second unit was operated by two men with identical first names. Harry and Harry processed my volunteer badge and parking permit. Their unit had the same paneling in its reception area, but behind the counter was a plaque that listed the winners of the annual hospital security dog contest. The same two dogs had alternated as first place finishers for the past eight years. Unlike with the first unit, I struggled to guess what message this unit might possibly be trying to signal. The virtues of redundancy? All I knew was that it left me wondering what criteria the hospital used in selecting people for positions, including the one I was about to fill.

The following day I attended an all-day orientation session for new and returning participants in the CPE program at an Episcopal church located in the affluent foothills of the city. Here I would get to meet the others the director had selected to provide spiritual care. The church had exquisite Spanish architecture with an elaborate array of courtyards. The room where the orientation was to be held was located just beyond the courtyards at the southwest corner of the complex, where a metal tray with coffee and napkins was set up outside the door. The room resembled a slightly enlarged and upgraded monastic cell with stucco walls, Saltillo floors, and a beamed ceiling that reached over ten feet. On the far wall was a faded photo of a collared Episcopal priest with a pair of glasses in hand, as if pausing from his studies. The room had fifteen chairs arranged in a tight circle, but it turned out that only six were needed. Except for the glow beneath the wooden door, the only light entering the room came through three deeply recessed windows on the south and east walls.

After I took a seat, the director entered and greeted me. He was dressed more casually than before, wearing jeans, an untucked denim shirt, and a string of beads on his right forearm. He also had two rings on his right hand that I had not noticed earlier (I later learned that he rotated them when saying a mantra).

When the other four program participants arrived, we sat in a semicircle and introduced ourselves. I was relieved to see that none of them, like the framed priest, wore a clerical collar. One was an effusive, middle-aged woman with mounds of blonde curls. She had worked under the director's supervision the year before and was back to finish her program, hoping to one day create a harp ministry in hospice settings. She was seated next to the director, and the two compared their beaded armlets. To her left was a slightly younger Catholic nurse who explained that she had decided to officially enroll in the program only five days earlier when she felt a calling from God to do so. Next to her was a woman of about the same age who had changed her name upon becoming a Buddhist priest. She wore a leg brace and shared her multiple health problems, as well as her experiences of living on an eighty-acre desert homestead where she planned to create a spiritual retreat. And next to her was a woman in her late fifties wearing thick glasses who had served as a local nun for the past thirty years. That we all deviated in some way from the stereotypical image of clergy suggested that the boundaries defining the profession had perhaps become more permeable since the time the Episcopal priest was photographed.

After I introduced myself, the director shared who he was. He had moved to town ten years ago and married last year, after having gone five years without any romantic relationship. He was currently reading a book on Crazy Horse and another on diets tailored to specific blood types. A former Episcopal priest, he now practiced kundalini yoga, which he claimed, among other things, enabled him to envision a peaceful parting of clouds while meditating. It was not a vision that I had ever experienced.

As the others, in turn, shared their spiritual tales, none of which resonated with me, my sense of incongruity grew. I was clearly in no danger of what social scientists call "going native" or identifying too closely with others and uncritically accepting their outlooks. My liberal Protestant background was more attuned to matters of social justice than to the kinds of mystical experiences the participants were sharing. At the same time, I was struck by their willingness to reveal deeply personal details of their lives, which softened me.

Following introductions, we spent time sharing our theories of pastoral care, assuming we came equipped with one, which I did not. After I made that awkward admission, we then ate an early lunch together at a Hare Krishna restaurant. When we returned to the church, we each acted out a different chaplain scenario to give the director an initial sense of our relational styles. The scenarios ranged from an immigrant's hysterical reaction to a grandmother's death (the Buddhist priest's) and a mom learning she had terminal cancer (the nurse's) to a woman in denial about her mother's death (the future harp chaplain's) and a rape victim being interrogated by a police officer (mine). The director judged my performance to be compassionate and thought I would excel at the program's Rogerian approach to pastoral counseling, which seeks to facilitate a client's self-discovery and actualization through empathetic and reflective listening. But he also felt I needed to "allow others to dwell longer in the emotional space I create for them," which I took to mean that I become uncomfortable not doing anything when hearing the depth of another individual's pain.

The director passed out thick notebooks containing detailed information on the CPE program, some of the possible reasons staff might call upon chaplains, and the hospital's clinical policies. He spent the most time discussing a section in the manual about recording our patient visits so that Medicare could reimburse the hospital for its pastoral care services. The program had averaged fourteen thousand annual visits for the past few years, but the director believed that if the program's participants would be more diligent about this matter, the count could be closer to twenty-five thousand, which supposedly would increase Medicare reimbursements. As I listened, I could not help but wonder whether the main reason he added me to the program was to ratchet up those numbers.

After skimming through other sections of the manual and giving us instructions about when and where we needed to go for our first workday at the hospital, the director concluded the session by telling a story. It was a winding narrative about a group of scholars who went to a holy man seeking answers to life's most difficult questions. The director described how this saintly person kept turning the scholars away, making them angrier and angrier, until at last the scholars stopped asking questions altogether and became open to experiencing the "truth."

I leaned back in my chair and thought, "I wonder which one of us he meant that for?" Whether he viewed this social scientist as chaplain material or not, I had no intention of checking my head in at the door.

It was not obvious to me who was cut out to perform the duties of a cleric in a public and highly scientized setting. Nor did it seem clear to the director of the hospital's chaplaincy services who interviewed me. Indeed, one of the puzzling developments in American religious life is that more and more spiritual care, which we defined earlier as affirming and upholding humans' transcendent quality, is now being provided by individuals outside the traditional boundaries of organized religion. As Sullivan (2014) explains, whereas in the past church and state were ideologically separated, members of the public now increasingly expect government establishments to promote spirituality as a universal aspect of humanity. This form of "spiritual governance" has long been practiced in the military, federal prisons, and the Veteran's Administration, where religious accommodations are mandated. But it is also becoming more the norm in other government-funded institutions like teaching hospitals. Though they are not required to endorse spirituality, these organizations often do so to maintain their legitimacy in the eyes of citizens who understand the spiritual as an expression of their true selves and hold public systems accountable for respecting and nurturing this facet of their personhood.

This development is especially important when viewed through the eyes of Weber, who suggested that religious authority is one of five mechanisms that will determine whether religion takes hold in modern, public life (Weber 1978). He predicted that as societies modernized, religion's influence would wane as clergy, theologians, and other religious elites were gradually pushed to the margins of most institutions. The expansion of spiritual responsibility into public arenas challenges that prediction—and yet, it is not clear exactly whose responsibility it will be. Who will do spiritual work on behalf of others? Who will have authority over spiritual matters? It could be traditional clergy. But others might also take on this role, be asked to assume it, or be assigned it as part of their job responsibilities. The hospital I studied voiced its support for integrating spirituality into care—but then eliminated its chaplaincy program. Who, then, was to take responsibility for spiritual care? Nurses are the hospital workers who have the most interaction with patients, and nursing as a profession has voiced a renewed commitment to care that respects patients' spirituality. Are nurses ready and able to fill this vacancy in religious authority and help ensure the survival of caritas?

This chapter addresses this question by asking whether nurses are willing to assume responsibility for the spiritual care previously provided by chaplains. Literature on secularization provides important insights into the fate of religious authority in modern societies, but it leaves some aspects of this issue open, namely, who besides clergy might perform this role. As discussed later, I found that the boundary separating chaplains and nurses was more porous than secularization scholars assume and that a significant number of nurses are prepared to perform or believe they are already performing clergy-like functions. This point suggests that caritas in the form of religious authority might stick, even in settings where professional clergy are absent, through the development of what Andrew Abbott (1988) calls craft-based authority. Before reviewing what secularization scholars have to say about religious authority and Abbott's research on this alternative form of authority, I provide background information on chaplains in teaching hospitals and the circumstances surrounding University Hospital's decision to terminate its chaplaincy program.

BACKGROUND

Teaching Hospitals and Chaplaincy

Historically, academic medical centers tasked chaplains with offering spiritual support to members of their church or denomination. These representatives of religion subsequently institutionalized their role through the creation of Clinical Pastoral Education (CPE) programs that train and certify individuals for ministry in hospital settings. But as more individuals, including some congregants, have distanced themselves from organized religion in self-identifying as "spiritual but not religious" and as psychotherapists and other professional groups have sought jurisdiction over "care of the soul" (Abbott 1988), chaplains' authority over spiritual matters has diminished to the point where it is no longer possible for them to claim "ownership" of the "transcendent" (Kendrick and Robinson 2000).

To win back some of the territory they have lost, hospital chaplains have lately sought to capitalize on the newly identified "need" for spirituality by claiming special expertise in that area. In doing so, they hope to transform chaplaincy from a peripheral service, applicable only to "religious" patients, into an integral element of patient care for all (Lee 2002, 339). Chaplains have also reasserted the distinctiveness of their role. As the hospital's director of chaplaincy services who hired me explained,

> In every culture, there does seem to be a need among humans to have a group of people who are trained and set apart for spiritual identity, purposes, and rituals. We, humans, need that type of symbolization. From the standpoint of human history, therefore, it does not look like just anybody could or should be a chaplain. Likewise, hospitals could not exist without some sort of boundary differentiation. It would be chaos. There needs to be a division of labor that distinguishes those charged with caring for patients' spiritual state from those responsible for other dimensions of their health.

Hospital chaplains' efforts to expand their base of operations and reclaim their authority, however, have proved largely ineffective. Believers and nonbelievers alike continue to view them as second-class clergy. Due to the ascendance of Christian nationalism, there is also considerable suspicion among those on the other end of the political spectrum about their place in public settings. Especially important is the fact that, as teaching hospitals have struggled to secure government funding, they have adopted efficiency-driven business models recommended by consulting firms like Press Ganey and West Hudson that only recognize evidence- and outcome-based authorities. This approach has forced chaplains to justify their presence by quantifying their "value for money," which is exceedingly difficult given the obscure goal of spiritual care. It also runs counter to the anti-intellectual orientation of CPE programs, only a handful of which conduct empirical research on their operations (VandeCreek 2003). As one chaplain resident at the hospital studied here put it, "We are asked to keep track of visits and referrals to show that staff members and patients need us. But not in terms of what happened in our encounters with them. I don't think that is easily measured. It goes beyond the scientific."

Religious Authority at University Hospital

As a result of hospitals being run more like businesses, chaplains' already marginalized roles are increasingly viewed as expendable. As the hospital's director of chaplaincy services put it, "If it came down to us and the guys who change the light bulbs, you know administration would let us go."[1]

Five months after making that statement, the director's fears were realized. The hospital announced that it would let go the entire staff of the clinical pastoral education program, which consisted of the full-time director, five full-time residents, and ten part-time interns. Largely because of the Balanced Budget Amendments of 1997, which reduced Medicare payments to teaching hospitals, the hospital had been forced to downsize over the years to the point where the chaplaincy program was no longer affordable. To be sure, eliminating a hospital's chaplaincy program is an extreme response to budget cuts. In fact, according to recent research (Handzo, Flannelly, and Hughes 2017), the percentage of hospitals employing chaplains increased from 2004 to 2016, regardless of a hospital's type (general versus specialist), funding mechanism (profit versus nonprofit), religious affiliation (affiliated versus nonaffiliated), and size (number of patients). This development was fueled in part by the growing emphasis on patient satisfaction and the popularity of palliative care. Still, the percentage of hospitals hiring board-certified chaplains—the kind that University Hospital had employed and trained—decreased by an estimated 15 percent across all hospital categories. In other words, hospitals are hiring chaplains, but they're hiring ones that have reduced training and expertise, likely because they can pay these chaplains less and allocate the savings to medical care.

In the weeks following the hospital's announcement that it would terminate its chaplains, there was considerable discussion among other hospital staff about who would fill the resulting void. When asked about the matter, one physician replied, "I am not sure that spiritual care is the exclusive role of chaplains . . . It's not the domain of any one profession." Another physician who specialized in oncology answered, "I am not sure it requires reassigning responsibilities. It is kind of like with kidney disease. I need to keep it in mind when treating a cancer patient who also has that condition. But that doesn't mean I need to have an expert on kidney disease always at my side. It just means I need to have a certain level of awareness. And so in some situations, I suppose you need a chaplain but in others it may not be necessary." Finally, a nurse said, "Well, nurses definitely see the patient, you know, the most. But yet they are the busiest, too . . . I mean, the nurses should take it into consideration, but it depends on the patient load that day. It's not going to be a priority. There are more life-threatening things that need to be taken care of . . . I can't think of a particular person who would take care of that [spiritual care]. I guess it would have to be everybody . . . or nobody."

How responsibility for spiritual care might be redistributed, if at all, in such a setting is key to the survival of caritas.

TOWARD A BETTER UNDERSTANDING OF RELIGIOUS AUTHORITY

Scholarship on Secularization

Secularization theory provides a useful way to approach this issue because it has much to say about religious authority. By the end of the twentieth century, about the same percentage of Americans believed in God, personal salvation, and the existence of heaven as in the beginning of the century. Some scholars interpret this persistence of belief as proof that modern society has entered a postsecular era. Secularization researchers, however, contend that, even though many Americans still subscribe to conventional religious doctrines, the capacity of religious authorities to regulate the behavior of laity has waned. They note that since the 1980s, over three-quarters of Americans believe that individuals should come to their moral values independent of what their church, synagogue, or mosque may say (Bellah et al. 1985).[2]

From these scholars' perspective, therefore, secularization is best understood not as declining religious beliefs, but the declining scope of religious authority as Weber had originally suggested (Dobbelaere 1988; Chaves 1994; Yamane 1997). Focusing on religious authority, these scholars contend, gets at the social—as opposed to individual—significance of religion. This approach is also consistent with sociological theorizing by Andrew Abbott (1988) about how professions compete to influence social life. According to this literature, professions establish themselves by marking out a particular sphere of work as their own jurisdiction, and this occupational territorialism can lead to rivalries between professional groups (Abbott 1988). Some jurisdictional claims constitute an attempted "invasion" of another profession's domain. In other cases, the claim is founded on the identification of a new "problem" that justifies the existence of the profession and its authority to address that problem.

Evidence of Declining Religious Authority

As proof that clergy's scope of authority is waning, secularization researchers cite evidence that within churches, ecclesiastical hierarchies are being flattened, clergy are being replaced in leadership positions by laity with valuable technical skills, and clergy's academic knowledge (theology) is being marginalized by an emphasis on operating churches more like corporations. For example, denominations today frequently choose professional administrators over bishops as CEOs (Chaves 1993; see also Dobblelaere 1988). In addition to this "internal secularization," scholars have documented the jurisdictional battles clergy have lost outside church walls—to medicine over the interpretation of illness, to psychiatry over everyday life problems, to social work over social welfare, and to lay teaching over control of the classroom (Abbott 1988).

Chaplains' recent relabeling of their work as "spiritual" is an example of how professions will seek to identify a new problem to reassert their authority. Chaplains have strategically deployed the concept of spirituality to extend the realm of their occupation's relevance to any patients' "belief system," regardless of their religious affiliation. But, as noted earlier, these efforts to claim jurisdiction over spiritual matters have been undercut, in large part, by a financial logic that deems them an unjustifiable expense. In the words of one chaplain resident,

> Do I think the demand for chaplains will increase or decrease over time? I think it has a little higher profile than it used to have. But as to whether chaplains' numbers will increase, if the medical funding keeps going the way it is, with HMOs managing more and more care, I think it will decrease. Not because there is not a place for it, but because nobody is willing to pay for it. There is a lot of cost cutting at this hospital. That trend is pretty national. Profit is the bottom line. This is a business.

In short, secularization suggests that as the forces of rationalization continue to transform the public sphere, religious authorities will be increasingly marginalized to the point that they eventually could be erased completely, removing one of the key cultural pillars of caritas in the process.

SECULARIZATION RECONSIDERED

Countertrends

As compelling as the evidence just noted might be, however, researchers who see secularization as declining religious authority fail to account for three important developments. First, as proponents of a "Religion on the Edge" perspective note, religious expressions have manifested themselves in several so-called secular venues (Cadge, Levitt, and Smilde 2011), politics being but one example. Evangelical networks permeate the upper reaches of the American political, educational, and media elite (Lindsay 2007). Likewise, progressive activists regularly invoke religious discourses and practices to mobilize many of their allies (Hondagneu-Sotelo 2008), including Christians and Jews who defend the labor rights of Latino immigrants.

Second, at the same time religious hierarchies have been gradually dismantled, so, too, have highly centralized structures elsewhere. During the early 1990s, for example, U.S. companies cut the layers of management by an astonishing 50 percent (Drucker 1995). In the process, Americans expressed their distrust of leadership across a range of institutions, including religion but also government, business, nonprofits, and the press (Rainie, Keeter, and Perrin 2019). The curtailing and questioning of authority, therefore, are by no means unique to religious organizations. Rather, they are characteristic of a larger trend throughout democratic societies.

Third, in the wake of this restructuring of organizational life, previously secularized corporations also appear to be going through a countervailing process of "sacralization" (Demerath 2000). Concerned about the demoralizing effects of corporate downsizing on their remaining workers, several businesses have begun experimenting with ways to create more "holistic" cultures that are sensitive to employees' spiritual needs. Firms have sponsored prayer breakfasts, Bible studies, and "vision quests," for example, to assist employees in their search for meaning and security at work, not to mention the ubiquitous mindfulness meditation programs sponsored by corporations (see Kucinskas 2018; Chen 2022). Ritual consultants, sacred designers, and soul-centered advertisers working for agencies with similar-sounding names—Sacred Design Lab, Ritual Design Lab, and Ritualist—have also emerged on the corporate scene to soften the cruelty of capitalism and make space for the soul. Major corporations like Taco Bell, Pizza Hut, and subsidiaries of Wal-Mart stores have even hired chaplains to help workers deal with nervous breakdowns, physical ailments, and family conflicts (Conlin 1999). In light of these and other changes, Laura Nash of the Harvard Business School and Ian Mitroff of the University of Southern California's Marshall School of Business have claimed that spirituality is "exploding in the workplace" (Nash 1999) and may be the "ultimate competitive advantage" (Mitroff and Denton 1999; see also Altman, Neal, and Mayhofer 2022). In 2020, *Forbes* magazine even went so far as to state that spirituality may be the hottest trend in the future workplace (Cappon 2020).

To be sure, it will take more than a spiritual uplift for workers to survive massive layoffs, and the number of downsized companies that can afford the long-term services of chaplains is probably quite small. Nonetheless, there seems to be a growing sentiment that spirituality warrants a place in the workplace, mirroring the spiritual care expected in government institutions (Sullivan 2014). For example, Oswick (2009) found that between the two 10-year periods ending in 1998 and 2008, the number of books on workplace spirituality increased threefold and the number of journal articles on the subject more than quadrupled.

This paradoxical turn to spirituality was not lost on the director of chaplaincy services at University Hospital. He commented,

> As institutions are more and more concerned about money, there is a huge non-denominational, non-church, non-sectarian movement in health care focused on spirituality and illness. . . . I think it is felt at the gut level and it seems to come from the realization that there are serious problems economically, relationally, and treatment wise with the allopathic model of medicine. The more technologically focused we become, the more a counter movement is growing defined by concerns about death and the search for meaning that is deeper than the physical, biological, reductionistic, hierarchical system we have created.

Just as corporations are advertising their new sensitivity to workers' spiritual needs, many of their leaders are also positioning themselves as legitimate providers of spiritual care—a trend that's reflected in the titles of some books on workplace spirituality, such as *The Healing Manager, On Becoming a Servant Leader*, and *Spiritual Leadership in Action*. These publications suggest how owners, executives, and other corporate leaders can become moral examples for their subordinates, in much the way that clergy have been to laity, through their displays of compassion and spiritual sensitivity. But they do not consider how responsibility for spiritual care might be transferred to other occupations, including frontline helping professions who directly care for the suffering.

CRAFT VERSIONS OF RELIGIOUS AUTHORITY

The Disappearing Boundaries Between Professions

This blurring of the boundaries between religious and secular occupations aligns with broader occupational trends. Andrew Abbott (1988, 65) explains that the "boundaries between professional jurisdictions tend to disappear in worksites, particularly in overworked worksites. There results a form of knowledge transfer that can be called workplace assimilation. Subordinate professionals, nonprofessionals, and members of related, equal professions learn on the job a craft version of a given profession's knowledge system." By craft version, he refers to certain tasks and forms of knowledge, such as spiritual care, that can be acquired by secondhand exposure to an occupation and be performed by others without formal certification. He suggests, therefore, that it's the work itself, not the workers' job title, that defines a profession's boundaries: "in the jurisdictional system of the workplace, it is the real output of an individual, not credentialed or non-credentialized status, that matters."

Scholars who have defined secularization as the declining scope of religious authority have drawn heavily on the work of Andrew Abbott. But Abbott's ideas about craft versions of authority have largely been ignored by these scholars. Part of the reason has to do with how they have defined religious authority. What distinguishes religious authority from other kinds of authority, they argue, is not the ends it pursues or the means it uses to get others to comply with its dictates, but rather that it bases its claims on a "language of the supernatural" (Chaves 1994, 756).

This definition is intuitively appealing in the sense that the "god talk" of clergy seems qualitatively different than the more rational language of administrators, economists, and other modern experts. Yet, upon closer examination, this definition is problematic. For it ignores the fact that it is precisely the language of the spiritual that is currently being invoked by both defenders and defectors of organized religion. As Roof explains (1993), those claiming to be "spiritual but not religious" use talk about spirituality to rescue what they perceive to be the real essence of religion from the institutional walls that have been built up around it.

Secularization scholars have also been slow in following through on their insight that using religion as the point of reference can blind one to sacralizing developments within secular organizations. As Demerath (2000) notes, researchers have used concepts like "invisible religion" (Luckmann 1967) and "folk religion" (Mathisen 1992) to suggest that the sacred is more than simply institutionalized religion. Yet they all use the latter as their basic point of reference. Hence, when deciding where to study the sacred, they ignore corporate settings that bear no overt relation to religion and are not described as "religious" by insiders or outsiders. Likewise, they presume that organizations that fall short of what constitutes a religious organization also fall short in providing sacred experiences. And they assume that when religion gives way to alternative meaning systems, a secularizing shortchanging necessarily occurs.

The Continuing Relevance of Religious Authority

To be fair, secularization scholars do not claim that there is a master trend toward religion becoming more differentiated from other spheres (see also Alexander 1990). Instead, they suggest that religion can become more or less differentiated depending on the time and place. For example, as mentioned earlier, within the United States, church and state have traditionally been ideologically separated, but in recent years government establishments have begun to promote spirituality as a universal aspect of humanity. However, secularization scholars do not push this important point far enough when considering the scope of religious authorities within organizations. Here the tendency is to describe secularization as a zero-sum game where religious authorities either win or lose in their jurisdictional battles with other professions. Applying the same logic to the case at hand, for example, they would ask whether hospital administrators considered clergy more expendable than other professions when forced to make budget cuts. What is missing from such a lifeboat approach, though, is a consideration of whether the survivors of downsizing are willing to assume the functions of jettisoned clergy. Or, to use Gorsky and Nelson's (2013) term, researchers fail to consider how individuals might "de-differentiate" themselves from religious professionals.

Lived religion scholars begin to explore this possibility in suggesting that the spiritual will remain important and even increase in social significance precisely because people can choose it voluntarily, on their own authority, as something they deeply value. But people often look for someone to assume spiritual authority—someone with special training or experience who can assume responsibility for spiritual care and guidance. And public institutions like hospitals fulfill obligations by assigning them to particular people as part of their job responsibilities. So, in hospitals and other public settings where spirituality is promoted, who will fill the space vacated by clerics?

METHODS

To begin to answer this question, surveyed nurses were asked their own opinions about assuming spiritual authority. As the earlier physicians' comments suggest, doctors tend to understand caregiving primarily in terms of technical competency and may regard spirituality as relevant but outside their scope of practice because it isn't part of their training (Cadge 2013).

But bedside nurses are in constant contact with patients, are trained to ask about patients' spirituality, and have been at the forefront of the spirituality in health care movement. At the same time, nursing is an especially demanding form of technical work, and in its efforts to be recognized as a true profession, it has tried to distance itself from the angelic stereotypes associated with it. To find out how nurses manage this tension, they were queried how willing and able they felt they were to perform the functions of displaced chaplains.

NURSES' OPINIONS ABOUT BECOMING
SURROGATE CHAPLAINS

Findings

To put their answers in context, it is important first to get a sense of how they feel about the ownership of spiritual concepts and about teaching hospitals as a potential space for spiritual experiences. As table 3.1 indicates, a quarter of the nurses used quasi-supernatural terms like "calling" to describe their work (see Raatikainen 1997). This finding suggests that the boundaries of religious authority created by the language of the supernatural are considerably more permeable than conceived by secularization scholars and therefore cannot be said to be "owned" by clergy.

TABLE 3.1
Nurses' opinions about spiritual care

Opinion	Percent
I consider my work a calling	25
I feel more spiritual at work than elsewhere	24
Nurses could provide most of the services by chaplains if nurses had more time and training	37
I would provide most of the services by chaplains if given more time and training	30
Chaplains are the best qualified hospital workers to address spiritual needs	50 (Disagree/Strongly Disagree)
All things considered, nurses provide more spiritual care to patients than chaplains	42

Note: Respondents were asked whether they Strongly Agreed, Agreed, Disagreed, or Strongly Disagreed with statements/opinions.

In keeping with Demerath's observation that individuals can have sacralizing experiences in nonreligious organizations (see Bailey 1998), nearly a quarter of nurses (24 percent) also said they feel "more spiritual at work than elsewhere." While other nurses felt more spiritual outside the hospital, most still viewed public teaching hospitals as a space that should be open to the spiritual. As reported in the previous chapter, a strong majority (72 percent) agreed that "hospitals should be concerned about the spirituality of their nurses," and nearly all (96 percent) disagreed or strongly disagreed that "promoting spirituality in hospitals is at odds with the real purpose of medicine."

As to nurses' opinions about taking over the spiritual care duties of chaplains, over a third (37 percent) felt that "nurses could provide most of the services by chaplains if nurses had more time and training," and nearly the same percentage (30 percent) said they themselves would actually do so. Nurses' willingness to take on this task did not vary much depending on their spiritual and religious identities. Over a fourth (28 percent) of "spiritual but not religious" nurses said they are willing to provide the same services as chaplains if given the time and training, which is only slightly less than the percent of "religious" nurses (37 percent) willing to perform this role. Clearly, not all nurses consider spiritual care the domain of chaplains, as some earlier research suggests (Ross 2006). Indeed, as other studies find, chaplains themselves often view nurses as "gatekeepers" to spiritual care and contestants in professional "turf wars" (Taylor and Trippon 2020).

Even more interesting, half (50 percent) of surveyed nurses disagreed or strongly disagreed with the statement that "chaplains are the best qualified hospital workers to address spiritual needs." *And a large minority of nurses (42 percent) went so far to agree with the statement "All things considered, nurses provide more spiritual care to patients than chaplains."* In other words, many nurses not only are willing to perform the functions of chaplains, but at some level think they already do. Importantly, this does not mean that nurses are necessarily arrogating religious authority to themselves. Rather, as Abbott (1988, 6) argues, "certain individuals in closely related professions end up knowing far more about a profession's actual work than do a fair number of its own practitioners." Or, as one chaplain resident and former nurse put it, "The other chaplains may not want to admit this, but nurses can do many of the same things they do."

Discussion

As previously mentioned, Abbott suggests that especially in overburdened work settings, where the boundaries between professions tend to become fuzzy, one profession will often learn and apply the skills of another. While public medical centers like University Hospital, which are chronically underfunded, can certainly be exhausting work environments, participants in the chaplaincy program also hinted at some other factors that might allow nurses to act as surrogates of chaplains. One was chaplains' marginalization in a scientific setting. A Catholic nun training to be a chaplain said, "The workers that least appreciate us are in ER. Oh yeah. They tolerate us and that's about it. They will put up with you and they are the ones who call if there is something really awful and they cannot control the situation and then they will call you. The workers who are slightly more appreciative are the ones dealing with terminal patients. The cancer ward, you know, that sort of thing. Or if there is a baby that is dying, and then you are called in to do a baptism." Similarly, another chaplain resident lamented, "I have tried to offer support to staff, some are receptive but a lot of them are like 'Chaplain? I don't need a chaplain.' And it is not always what they say, sometimes it is just the look on their faces. So, I just let them be."

Another factor possibly contributing to nurses' assimilation of chaplains' role is that they have more regular contact with patients. As one chaplain resident explained, and I also found to be true,

> Many nurses here are very caring and provide a lot of comfort in ways we cannot because they are with the patients so much more. I'm thinking of one nurse on 5E [Medical Surgery] who is very interested in the spiritual aspects of nursing. She would draw me aside and tell me about her interactions with different patients, their spiritual backgrounds, and how she was able to connect with them. And many times she would kind of give me entrée into their lives because she had already been talking to them about their faith. It told me some nurses can really get close to patients.

Yet another possible reason that chaplains' spiritual care might be assimilated by nurses, most of whom identify as women, has to do with the feminine nature of such care. The director of chaplaincy services alluded to this possibility in describing his approach to chaplaincy. "I don't divorce the psychological from the spiritual. According to Erickson, a child's psychological development begins when he or she learns either to trust or distrust their caregiver. That is, it all boils down to the interaction with the mother so that a child either feels sufficiently loved or not. So that initial and decisive stage involves a strong ingredient of maternal care. . . . I will often say to chaplain trainees, one way to think about pastoral care is that you are trying as a professional to be a 'good enough mother.'"

CONCLUSION

In this chapter, we drew on secularization research to better understand nurses' willingness to assume responsibility for the spiritual care of their patients. While this scholarly literature helped us understand clergy's shrinking sphere of influence in modern society, it hasn't paid much attention to spirituality outside of churches and other religious institutions—places generally considered secular. And in fact, more and more people have become interested in spirituality as hierarchical religious institutions have flattened out and reduced their ranks, leaving space for others to act as providers of spiritual care.

Scholars have not yet explored this clergy-like behavior, even though many recognize that in overburdened work environments, professional boundaries often become blurred, leading members of one profession to assimilate the knowledge and tasks of another (Abbott 1988). We considered some of the reasons that secularization researchers have failed to act on this insight and their relevance to nurses' opinions about acting as surrogates of chaplains. This, in turn, allowed us to develop a more nuanced understanding of how the first of the five cultural mechanisms identified by Weber—authority—enables spirituality to "stick" in scientific settings and thus enhances caritas's chances of survival.

Results from our survey of nurses suggest that even if traditional religious authority does decline, religious ethics like caritas might still survive because authority over them will transfer to specific others. These findings are actually consistent with secularization scholars' writings on differentiation. They suggest that instead of "religion" broadly, and religious authority broadly, we get religion subdivided into particular ethics, practices, and perspectives that become the responsibility of different groups—in this case, nurses acquire responsibility or authority for caritas.

Similarly, as many religious organizations are becoming more internally secularized, many nonreligious organizations seem to be going through a countervailing process of "sacralization" (Demerath 2000). University Hospital may be one such organization; its leaders have certainly taken steps to introduce spirituality into its corporate culture under the banner of "holistic care"; at the same time, the hospital ended its chaplaincy program. Secularization theorists like Chaves help make sense of the end of the chaplaincy program but couldn't predict that the hospital would continue to emphasize spirituality in the wake of this program's demise. Abbott's work, meanwhile, helps makes sense of the hospital's transfer of spiritual duties to its nursing staff. This chapter brings these two lines of thought together to argue that secular settings like hospitals may be fertile ground for craft versions of religious authority to take root. Even as traditional religious leaders—chaplains—lose authority, that authority devolves onto other workers—in this case, scientifically trained nurses.

This notion does not imply that all clergy will eventually be supplanted. As others have demonstrated, religious figures like chaplains have not only established a presence in secular settings like the military and prisons (Sullivan 2014) but are also reinventing themselves as humanizing agents in others, including fast-food restaurants, retail stores, and seaports (Cadge and Skaggs 2019). However, because of the open-ended nature of their care work and the public's strong trust in them, frontline helping professionals like nurses are likely to come under pressure to perform clergy-like functions, especially when dealing with clients experiencing existential crises and during historical periods when clerical hierarchies are being leveled.

Of course, this study is not the first to observe religious authority being laicized within organizations. There are numerous examples of contemporary churches (Calvary Chapel, Hope Chapel, the Vineyard Fellowship) that have rigorously applied the principle of the "priesthood of all believers." This study is unique in suggesting that a similar phenomenon might also take place within secular organizations attempting to reintroduce spirituality.

It remains unclear what the long-term consequences of such cases will be, but they promise to provide new insight into the (de)secularization process during an age when authority structures are being downsized and caring tasks reassigned. They may reveal that craft and professional versions of religious authority operate concurrently and that the development of the former cannot be sustained without the presence of the latter. It could also be that as willing as some laity are to provide the services of religious professionals, there is little demand for them to do so because they lack the symbolism associated with the latter. Or it may be that as organizations retrench and workers are further demoralized, more nonprofessionals will be encouraged to work alongside religious professionals, resulting in a net increase in spiritual care.

In addition, studying craft versions of religious authority would help us better understand whether clergy or laity are the chief "carryovers" from one religious movement to the next (see Taylor 1989). What explains, for example, the resurgence of religion in the wake of secular nationalism in the third world and communism in Europe? If it's true, as Dobbelaere argues, that religion is periodically edged out of public life and then brought back in, as was the case in these regions of the world, then it makes sense to examine both official religious authorities and quasi-religious authorities to determine which people in which positions are the "sacralizers" and which are the "secularizers" (Dobbelaere 1981, 61). And studying these actors would further our understanding of how individuals find role models and moral direction in an age of "lite heroes," when the morality of clergy and other institutional leaders are increasingly questioned (see Wuthnow 1993).

Americans have an insatiable appetite for celebrity and the sensational, so when public attention turns to religion, it tends to fixate on religion's saints and villains. In this context, the ordinary people who uphold the sacred and perform craft versions of spiritual authority tend to be hidden in plain view—as I came to realize as a hospital chaplain and again as a transplant donor.

Our flight to Pittsburgh lands on Friday at 1:00 A.M. As we shuttle to the terminal and my expectations begin to rise, I remind myself that even if I am deemed an acceptable donor, there is no guarantee that the procedure will be successful. The immune system lacks the ability to distinguish friendly from unfriendly foreign tissue. Rejection is a part of the transplant process and must be controlled for the transplant to work. In the years leading up to my dad's diagnosis and after, tremendous advances in immunosuppression therapy have been made. But surgeons still cannot promise that the graft will take. Nor is it clear who in

the hospital will be responsible for helping us, visitors from an outside state, should the surgery fail.

From the airport, we take a cab to the Family House, a thirty-nine-room facility for the families of patients recovering from or waiting for a transplant and, in our case, patients and their potential living donors. As Lee Gutkind (2014) explains, Family House was opened in 1983 after a $1.2 million renovation, remodeling and connecting two existing and vacant Victorian houses with stained glass, beamed ceilings, and oak banisters. Before Family House, the families of patients stayed in motel rooms or, if that was beyond their means, in patients' hospital rooms, curled up in chairs in lounges and waiting rooms, or sprawled along the walls in hospital corridors.

As we are walking up to the building's front porch, a weary middle-aged couple emerges from behind its French doors, pushing a teenage girl in a wheelchair. While holding the door for us, they explain that their daughter had a transplant several months earlier but must now go through the entire process again. They are en route to the transplant center, having just been notified that a possibly suitable cadaver has become available. Like many other visitors at the Family House, this couple offer us support and practical advice throughout our stay. Weeks from now, they will even write to say they are thinking of us three days after their daughter eventually dies due to postoperative complications.

After settling into our room at the Family House, my dad and I walk two blocks that same day to the University of Pittsburgh Medical Center's transplant center, where we undergo a series of tests to determine whether our livers are compatible and we are both capable of surviving the procedure. The process is extensive, understandably so given that liver transplantations are expensive and technically difficult. My testing begins by meeting with a nurse, who reviews my medical records to confirm that I have never suffered from diabetes, hypertension, cancer, vascular disease, or untreated fungal, bacterial, or viral infections, or was ever a drug or alcohol abuser. If individuals have any of these conditions, they are immediately disqualified as donors.

Having passed that initial hurdle, I am taken to a blood lab, where nearly two dozen vials of blood are drawn. Next, I am led to a surgical room, where a nurse takes tissue samples from me to determine whether my and my dad's blood types are well matched (organs are usually not transplanted across the ABO blood type grouping) and to assess the vitality of my organs. During the biopsies, a needle is inserted in my liver. It's painless but makes a disconcerting popping sound as it penetrates the outer layer of the organ. A CT scan of my liver's anatomy is then taken in another room to gauge my liver's size and identify any abnormalities that might interfere with the success of the transplant. The transplant team also examines my liver through ultrasound to create a picture of the liver and surrounding organs. The effectiveness of my liver as a refinery is evaluated by injecting me with a special dye (indocyanine green test) and measuring how it is processed and cleared. An endoscopy is conducted that involves passing a lighted tube through the esophagus and stomach to see if varicose veins, which can cause fatal hemorrhaging during surgery, are present.

I next undergo a series of pulmonary function tests to measure lung capacity and ability to tolerate a lengthy operation under anesthesia. Living donor liver transplants can require up to eighteen hours. Finally, I am interviewed by a medical social worker to assess whether I have been coerced by others to donate my liver and am prepared for the possibility that I either will have failed some step in the evaluation process or the transplant procedure does not work. She reminds me that the body's automatic rejection of organs transplanted into it can be controlled but not entirely prevented by new immunosuppression drugs.

As I am led by a nurse out of the social worker's office and down one of the hospital hallways, I ponder how an organ can reject the very graft that could grant it life, what kind of compromise is necessary for the two to coexist. The nurse steps aside to make room for a large family when we walk past the hospital's chapel. Perhaps it is a late addition or was there from the beginning and corridors were later built up around it, but the chapel feels like an interruption in the hallway's otherwise orderly and mechanical flow, reminiscent of the one I frequented as a chaplain back in Tucson that also seemed awkwardly situated in its hospital. Glancing through its stained-glass images of skies, trees, and running streams, I see what looks like an unlit multipurpose room filled with about a dozen folding, wooden chairs. Except for what I gather is a book containing written prayers on a table against the far wall, the chapel is shorn of all religious symbolism, as was the case with its Tucson counterpart. As a patient, I am struck by its neutrality and the silent, tenuous truce it conveys. But perhaps because I relied on nurses for guidance during my time as a chaplain, I also cannot help but notice something else. As she passes the chapel, the nurse, dressed in a bright, multicolored blouse, almost looks like an extension of the brilliant, many-hued light coming through the decorative glass. It is an evocative and reassuring reminder that authority over spiritual care is not bounded but can stretch to the edges of religion and beyond.

Chapter Four

SECOND-GUESSING TALK
ABOUT SPIRITUALITY

Soon after I entered the chaplaincy program and met the other staff members, I began to ask myself how to broach the topic of spirituality with other hospital workers and patients. This question of how to talk about spirituality has everything to do with the survival of caritas: if the idea that strangers possess a universal, transcendent quality is to "stick" in public life, we need to be able to discuss that quality and understand what conditions are necessary for people to feel comfortable talking about it. Within our little "God squad," the spiritual was nearly always on the table for conversation, but it was unclear whether others in the hospital would welcome talk about spirituality. Without this clarity, I resorted to trying to read people's minds and intuitively assess their comfort with the topic—and I regularly missed the mark.

The Monday after our orientation session, the other program participants and I gathered in the hospital's chapel, where we met the staff chaplain and the full-time chaplain interns who were starting their second year of the Clinical Pastoral Education (CPE) program. I expected this experienced group to be less like our own and more like the photo of the Episcopal priest I had seen at the orientation, whose professionalism and religiosity were unmistakable. But like us, most of them were not especially "professional." Nothing about them stood out as clergy material. Over time, though, as we regularly met, I came to realize how, despite all appearances, this group and ours seemed to be cut from the same cloth as the priest in that we shared a deep interest in the spiritual. This realization, in turn, made it easier to invoke the language of the numinous in one another's presence.

The staff chaplain was a married man in his mid-thirties with a stout, bearish appearance who used to be an amateur baseball catcher. He wore a Promise Keepers badge (Promise Keepers is an Evangelical men's movement) just beneath his hospital ID on his left lapel and belonged to a small Free Methodist church, where he oversaw kitchen cleanup after the church's potlucks.

The oldest of the chaplain interns was also married—a mild-mannered man who seemed to be in his late fifties and had a bald head and a round, fleshy face. He had been raised Baptist but now belonged to a local, nondenominational megachurch. He wanted to join his church's staff and hoped that his training at the hospital would help him get hired. The staff chaplain later told me that of the four interns, he was the most trustworthy and the best at keeping confidences.

The next-oldest chaplain was a thin, silver-haired man in his mid-forties who had a master's degree in Buddhist meditation and lived with his wife in a small, nearby desert town. He was vegan, well read in philosophy, and openly skeptical about claims of miraculous healing. Frustrated with his work as an accountant, he was hoping the CPE program would help him find a new career path. The week before I joined the group, he had talked an armed patient out of committing suicide.

The youngest chaplain interns were both women. The older of the two was single, in her early thirties, and had dark, glossy bangs that barely touched the top of her glasses. In keeping with her simple attire—a blue cotton t-shirt and plain slacks—she was a lifetime Quaker who rejected the idea that her tradition was a "religion." She came across as very thoughtful and gentle in her interactions with others. Others considered her one of the two quietest people in the program (the other one being myself).

The other woman was also single. She was glamorous, had long, flowing brunette hair, and looked like she was in her twenties. She wore flamboyant, tropical dresses and was an accomplished Flamenco guitarist, and she was currently pursuing a career as a hospital counselor. She did not say whether she had a religious affiliation, but she had a master's degree in world religions and mentioned dating a physician intern who was studying Jainism.

My group's participation in the CPE program was limited to six months of unpaid, part-time work, which consisted of four hours of training each week and twelve hours of clinical visitations. A good portion of our training was spent with the full-time chaplain and chaplain interns. Training took place every Tuesday from 1 to 5 P.M. and included three seminars: theory seminars led by the CPE director that addressed various pastoral, ethical, and health care concerns from an interdisciplinary perspective with special emphasis on a Rogerian approach to counseling that uses reflective listening to create opportunities for patients to develop a sense of self-determination; case seminars in which we reviewed and critiqued one another's case reports of pastoral visits; and interpersonal relations seminar that utilized the group to explore personal and professional issues related to the chaplaincy role as well as our interactional styles. We also had individual supervision where participants would meet one on one with the CPE director to evaluate their growth and progress toward their learning goals. Clinical visitations usually took place one day a week after the chaplain interns completed their morning shifts and lasted from 6 P.M. to 6 A.M. During that time, one of us would be the only on-call chaplain in the hospital. We slept and waited for calls in what looked like a large storage closet that had a small desk and single bed with plastic pillow coverings.

Before taking on this role, we part-time students spent two weeks shadowing a chaplain intern. While the purpose of this exercise was to familiarize us with hospital staff and protocol, I was frequently distracted by patients themselves and their physical conditions. My fixation on pain, pus, blood, and other graphic sights and the creeping unease they engendered grew to the point where I sometimes wondered whether medical staff were even aware of what ordinary people would find to be disgusting and horrifying. For example, I was once in the ER, where a young physician was trying to console a former nurse whose deceased mother lay on a table between them. The former nurse was upset about how impersonally she and her family had been treated by staff. She pointed out the difference between sympathy (a largely cognitive state) and empathy (a deeply emotional one). The physician shared that she, too, knew the pain of losing a parent and did in fact feel for the nurse and her family. The two hugged. What most captured my attention about the situation, though, was something that I thought the physician failed to notice—a foot with only three toes sticking out from underneath the sheet covering the deceased mother. How could the physician not see and comment to the daughter about this grotesque object? It turned out she had noticed. When the daughter left and the physician was summarizing the case in her microrecorder, she mentioned that judging from the patient's left foot, she had likely been a diabetic. What struck me as bizarre was prosaic to her.

Unfortunately, my failure to concentrate on how chaplains approached and interacted with patients showed when I eventually took over as the single on-call chaplain. It was then that I discovered how, outside our chaplaincy circle, comfort with God talk cannot be assumed and is subject to misinterpretation. I was to begin my rounds by visiting patients scheduled for surgery later that evening. I slowly entered the room of my first patient, an elderly man who had been admitted for the second time that week. Instead of gently knocking on the door as I had been instructed, I suspected that he might not hear well because of his age, so I announced in a louder-than-usual voice that I was tonight's chaplain. But I misjudged—my booming announcement that a chaplain was in the room startled an already anxious patient. He immediately clutched his chest and gasped that no one had told him that he might not survive a knee replacement. When he calmed down, he demanded to see my chaplain's ID.

These and other early forays into chaplaincy impressed upon me how difficult it can be to read people's comfort with spiritual talk in settings like hospitals, where death and suffering are part of the normal routine.

Spirituality can be an awkward topic to discuss and therefore subject to second-guessing. Because it's such a sensitive topic, people are often unsure whether they should broach the subject in conversation. Often, they're forced to act on a hunch—and sometimes a blind one—about other people's comfort with the topic.

Conventional wisdom suggests that for communities to exist, their members must share a common language. But Max Weber, the father of interpretive sociology, questioned whether a shared language is sufficient to create shared understandings (Weber 1958c). He thought that another ingredient was necessary for a community to form and grow: people must believe that their speech will be comprehended and welcomed by others (Tada 2018). If he is right, then it is not enough for hospitals to promote spirituality; talk about spirituality among nurses must be an understood and welcomed part of their work culture. Nurses will only talk about spiritual matters if they think other nurses will welcome such talk.

During my time as a chaplain intern, I was struck by the fact that despite working in an environment where existential crises are commonplace, nurses rarely seemed to discuss spirituality among themselves. As one nurse shared with me, "The spiritual aspects of our work are so blatantly obvious that they are almost intolerable to talk about. I'm able to but most nurses are not. They simply won't open up." And yet, as we discovered in the previous chapters, the vast majority of nurses at University Hospital are personally interested in spirituality, and many feel they are actually more skilled than chaplains at addressing patients' spiritual needs. This begs the question: how accurately do nurses perceive one another's discomfort in discussing spiritual matters, and under what conditions are they most likely to be wrong? This is an important issue because if caritas is to become part of public life, frontline care workers like nurses must perceive one another as comfortable using spiritual language, it being one of the channels that Weber suggested can transmit religious ideals like caritas. If not, this religious ethic will likely not register and be subject to second-guessing. To begin to address this issue, I turn to literature on pluralistic ignorance, which suggests some of the reasons that group members might avoid talking about matters that are important to them and how we might conceptualize and measure the type of second-guessing that often ensues.

HOW PLURALISTIC IGNORANCE CAN HELP US UNDERSTAND WHY NURSES MIGHT NOT DISCUSS SPIRITUALITY

Social life depends on individuals being able to take into account the thoughts and feelings of others. When we decide to bring up a topic, express a view, or raise a question, we do so based on what we believe others are thinking and whether they share our opinions. But the judgments on which we predicate our social behavior sometimes turn out to be wrong (e.g., Allport 1924), even judgments about the opinions of our peers. For example, students may hesitate to ask questions because they are under the false impression that their classmates understand the course material better than themselves. Individuals living in an all-white community may mistakenly assume that they are the only residents in their neighborhood opposed to racial housing segregation (Greeley and Sheatsley 1971; Schuman, Steeh, and Bobo 1985).

Scholars have labeled these instances of pluralistic ignorance—situations where a majority (plurality) of individuals perceive that most of their peers think differently than themselves when, in fact, their attitudes are similar (hence, they are ignorant of what is actually going on in others' minds). When sociologists first began studying the phenomenon, they attributed this misperception to group members' lack of mutual visibility (Greeley and Sheatsley 1971; Schuman, Steeh, and Bobo 1985), suggesting that pluralistic ignorance occurs when group members are physically separated from one another and therefore have to guess at what they are thinking. Psychologists subsequently challenged this explanation. Noting that pluralistic ignorance often occurs where group members can readily observe one another, such as in a classroom, they suggested that pluralistic ignorance is a result of taking people's public behavior as an indicator of their private thoughts and feelings. According to psychologists, because perceptions rest on behavioral observation, pluralistic ignorance is actually more, not less, likely when mutual observability is high (Miller and McFarland 1991).

The Relevance of Pluralistic Ignorance to Spiritual Talk

Early on in this research project, there were hints that a similar phenomenon might be preventing hospital nurses from discussing spirituality among themselves. When asked during presurvey interviews whether the topic of spirituality ever came up in their work, nurses who said that it did would almost invariably cite conversations they had with patients. For example, one nurse answered that "we definitely hear from patients about their interest in spirituality. And it's really interesting, too, because once you give them a little permission to talk about such things, they really open up. But it is not that surprising when you consider their entire experience in the hospital is personal in nature. If they tell us about their bowel movements without batting an eye, why should we be surprised if they share their opinions about religion, God, etc.?" Survey results also confirmed that spirituality is a topic broached by many patients. Nearly half (48 percent) of nurses agreed or strongly agreed with the statement "The topic of spirituality often comes up with my patients."

In contrast, nurses rarely referenced a discussion about spirituality they had with a coworker. Indeed, some seemed puzzled when asked how comfortable their fellow nurses were discussing the subject. As one nurse put it, "I don't know. I suppose more nurses would be open to talking about spirituality than not, whether they had actually . . . well, I'll take that back. Did you say talk about? I am not so sure." Others expressed their frustration at not being able to converse about spirituality with other nurses. When asked how easy it is for her colleagues to talk about this matter, one nurse replied,

> It would probably be the most difficult thing for them to discuss. I'm very open about my spirituality. Religious etiquette requires people to follow a certain track and not impose their beliefs on others. There is nothing wrong with that. I respect that. But until an individual is willing to open up their perspective and realize, for example, that this Jesus they are worshipping isn't this white man they have seen in a picture, that his skin was almost as dark as a black man, that he didn't speak English, that his name, Jesus, was probably pronounced completely different, and that he believed in YAHWEH, Jehovah, . . . until they do those sorts of things, they shut themselves off from a real conversation about spirituality.

Granted, she was referring to just one type of spiritual understanding that is popular among white evangelicals and her idea of a "real conversation" might have been more confrontational than others', but her statement nonetheless speaks to the silence surrounding the topic of spirituality among her peers. Her suggestion that this silence is due to "religious etiquette" also echoes the widely shared belief that some topics cannot be discussed in public, especially in scientific settings, because they make others uncomfortable. But, as will be revealed, not only are most nurses comfortable discussing spirituality, but the perception that their fellow nurses are not also varies greatly across units within the hospital. This suggests that something other than good manners is at work.

To illuminate this situation, we will examine some of the social factors that may explain why some nurses think that their fellow nurses are uneasy discussing spirituality when, in fact, that is not the case. What, besides religious etiquette, might lead to this perception? Pluralistic ignorance is one answer: if most nurses think their peers aren't comfortable discussing spirituality, they'd be likely to keep their thoughts to themselves. The next section develops this possibility by looking at how scholars have defined and analyzed pluralistic ignorance. I build on this work to suggest some of the conditions under which pluralistic ignorance might come into play in nurses' conversations about spirituality (or lack thereof): in what kinds of settings, at what times, among which nurses, do nurses misperceive one another's willingness to engage in spiritual talk? Answers to this question will provide fresh insight into the conditions under which caritas as a language, another of the mechanisms mentioned by Weber for transmitting values, is likely to take root in scientized work environments.

UNPACKING PLURALISTIC IGNORANCE AND HOW IT COULD PREVENT SPIRITUAL TALK

The Nature and Meaning of Pluralistic Ignorance

While considerable research has been done on pluralistic ignorance, there remains much confusion about its nature and meaning. And so it is important that we address these issues if we are to fully appreciate how pluralistic ignorance might shape the likelihood that nurses talk about spirituality. As social psychologists Deborah Prentice and Dale Miller (1993, 161) point out, the term "pluralistic ignorance" is actually something of a misnomer. Where this phenomenon is present, group members are not, in fact, ignorant in the sense of being stupid. Instead, they think they know another's private sentiments, but they are really mistaken. Nor is the so-called ignorance truly pluralistic: it is an error that individuals make in judging the sentiments of the plurality or misperceiving what is the majority opinion (Shamir and Shamir 1997). In addition, pluralistic ignorance is not a condition that does or does not exist (Korte 1972, 579). Rather, it is a phenomenon that varies in severity. At one end of its continuum are instances of *relative* pluralistic ignorance, or situations where individuals slightly over- or underestimate the majority opinion. At the other end are examples of *absolute* pluralistic ignorance, or situations where persons misperceive the majority opinion on an issue to be the minority view (or vice versa).[1] Of primary interest to this study are the latter, absolute types.

Scholars also distinguish between two forms of group ignorance. With out-group ignorance, individuals share erroneous beliefs about groups to which they do not hold membership. With in-group ignorance, members of the same group hold false ideas about one another. We will be focusing on the latter, more surprising variety of pluralistic ignorance.

Scholars note further that pluralistic ignorance is distinct from two related phenomena—the false consensus effect (the tendency of people to overestimate their similarity to others) and the false uniqueness effect (the tendency to underestimate self-other similarity). The chief difference is that whereas false consensus and false uniqueness effects refer just to the misperceptions of a single individual, pluralistic ignorance refers to situations where misperceptions are widely shared by members of a group and both false consensus and uniqueness effects can be present (O'Gorman 1986).

Given the confusion surrounding the nature and meaning of the term, what has been traditionally called pluralistic ignorance might be more appropriately labeled a mutually misperceived norm. Regardless of the conceptual tag used, however, the biggest problem surrounding the study of the phenomenon has been getting a better empirical handle on its causes.

Past Research on Pluralistic Ignorance

Having reviewed some of the difficulties researchers have had in conceptualizing pluralistic ignorance, we next consider some of the shortcomings of past research on the subject. Here, too, we need to address these limitations if we are to completely grasp how this phenomenon may prevent nurses from conversing about spiritual matters.

Although interest in shared misperceptions goes back as far as Plato's consideration of false opinions, pluralistic ignorance was first identified as a technical problem in the social and behavioral sciences by an American psychologist named Floyd Allport, who coined the term nearly eighty years ago (Allport 1924; see also O'Gorman 1986). Allport (1924, 320) noted that while a requisite of social life is knowledge of "how others habitually feel and think concerning various matters," individuals often do not have access to such information. As a result, those who hold a majority opinion tend to falsely assume that most others share their views. Allport feared that these false impressions could be manipulated and used to control individuals in undesirable ways. His treatment of pluralistic ignorance, however, was fairly cursory. He noted the importance of the phenomenon, provided examples of it, but did not formally analyze it. Indeed, Allport saw nothing unusual in the fact that individuals can be wrong in their perceptions of others.

The topic of pluralistic ignorance was all but ignored for forty years after Allport's seminal study. Beginning in the late 1960s, however, sociologists became curious about the phenomenon when they stumbled on an even more ironic form of it in which a majority falsely imputed their opinions to a minority. They discovered, for example, that although most whites rejected segregationist policies following the passage of the Civil Rights Act, they were under the false impression that only a few whites thought like themselves (Greeley and Sheatsley 1971; Schuman, Steeh, and Bobo 1985). Similarly, sociologists found that a majority of elderly individuals thought they were financially secure but assumed that only a minority of the aged population felt the same (O'Gorman 1980, 1986). In trying to explain these misperceptions, sociologists turned to Robert Merton, who himself wrote very little about the subject but suggested that pluralistic ignorance is "a frequently observed condition of a group which is so organized that mutual observability of its members is slight" (Merton 1968, 431).

Psychologists later attacked sociologists' explanation by citing examples in which group members were ignorant of a norm even when in the presence of one another. They noted, for instance, that students frequently do not ask questions in class because they mistakenly believe that others are less confused than themselves and that bystanders often do not respond to emergency situations because they misperceive that others are less concerned than themselves. Based on such examples, psychologists concluded that "Merton's generalization is fundamentally wrong" (Miller and McFarland 1991, 290) and that pluralistic ignorance is actually enhanced by mutual observability.

More recently, sociologists have conceded that pluralistic ignorance is possible where mutual observability is high. They note that not only can false ideas be shared among individuals who are physically separated and do not know each other, but they can also be shared by individuals who participate together in small social systems and do know one another. For example, Eliasoph and Lichterman (2003; Eliasoph 1998) document the presence of pluralistic ignorance among assembled peers in their studies of political discourse. Contrary to the notion that persons are too small-minded or ignorant to converse about political matters, they show that most individuals relish such conversations with their peers. However, individuals frequently refrain from broaching the topic of politics when in the company of their social equals because they are under the false impression that their social equals do not welcome such talk. Citizens who are quite interested in and knowledgeable of political issues, therefore, often work hard at not discussing such matters publicly. They censor their talk either because they perceive they would violate existing speech norms or because the issues themselves are simply too vast in scope for individuals to influence. Thus they inadvertently create "spirals of silence" (Noelle-Neumann 1993) and cultures of political avoidance that can be mistaken for apathy. Elia-soph and Lichterman suggest further that unpopular speech norms may surround several topics that group members privately consider to be of ultimate importance, including religion. And such norms may be present in a variety of small social systems, like work and volunteer organizations, where peers often come together.

Is Second-Guessing Spiritual Talk Solely Due to Physical Proximity?

As mentioned earlier, Weber suggests that conversation plays a crucial role in society, that we need a shared language to create and maintain the reality of everyday life (see also Berger and Luckmann 1966; Ammerman 2014; Wuthnow 2011). He also conceded that as societies have modernized, it has become more difficult for individuals to rely on traditional religious languages to discuss the ultimate concerns they share. Scholars differ, though, over whether such languages might be transformed to better express and generate transcendent understandings.

Secularization researchers suggest that religious talk in general has become obsolete. Concepts like the soul, they point out, are increasingly expunged from scientific conversation. And where such talk has survived, it has often been a source of division and a threat to progress, most obviously in the case of religious extremism. More optimistic scholars contend that contemporary talk about spirituality (Roof 1999; Besecke 2013) is highly compatible with rationality because it's often less dogmatic than it is *reflexive*, which in this context means that people who talk about spirituality reflect on their spiritual ideas as one set of ideas among many other valid possibilities. People who practice a reflexive spirituality are open to the possibility of belief and, at the same time, willing to question the grounds of faith. This language deemphasizes the concept of an immortal soul but retains the idea of the sacredness of the person (Joas 2013).

In today's religiously pluralistic world, many people see *spirituality* as a neutral word that enables people from different faith perspectives and people who don't identify with any particular religious tradition to find common ground. In a society where religion is often associated with division and conflict, the language of spirituality makes it easier for people to exchange ideas about the sacred and to transition from small talk to deeper conversations about the supreme worth of individuals (Bender 2003). More generally, as lived religion scholars suggest, such talk makes it easier for people to explain their faith to others (Ammerman 2014).

Literature on pluralistic ignorance would suggest that there is an element of truth to both arguments. On the one hand, individuals may share a private interest in spirituality and welcome conversation about this ultimate concern. On the other hand, they may refrain from engaging in such talk because it is perceived as a violation of modern speech norms that privilege science. And such misperceptions are especially likely to occur where like-minded actors are gathered together in the same physical locale.

Still, extant research on pluralistic ignorance can only take us so far in our understanding of the misperceptions surrounding spiritual talk within small social systems. Despite the strong possibility that other factors besides physical proximity may influence the transparency of group norms, scholars have failed to suggest what these other hidden obstacles might be and test their effects. As a result, there remains a strong tendency to attribute the lack of public talk about topics like spirituality to conversational taboos.

To better understand why caritas as discourse may not materialize in modern, clinical settings, in the next section I draw on three strands of literature that suggest what factors besides etiquette might explain why nurses working at the same hospital would refrain from discussing spirituality.

Other Potential Sources of Pluralistic Ignorance

Eliasoph and Lichterman's (2003) research on speech norms points to one possible source of pluralistic ignorance. It suggests that the more prominent an issue is on a group's agenda, the less likely it will be subject to pluralistic ignorance. That is, if a topic is regularly brought up at official group assemblies, members will have more opportunities to observe others' reactions to it and gather more accurate information on their opinions.

Literature on the cultures of organizations (Martin 1992) hints at another set of factors that condition individuals' ability to accurately gauge norms. According to it, coworkers have a more difficult time assessing the majority's opinion in larger task units or where there are more opinions that must be taken into account. The position a worker occupies within an interpersonal network may also be more or less conducive to forming intimate relationships, which influence the depth, quality, and accuracy of information that is exchanged.

Finally, studies of workplace performance allude to still other factors that may color perceptions. Appelbaum and Batt (1994) argue that more technologically demanding activities can alienate individuals from their feelings as well as from those of their colleagues. Research by Hochschild (1983) on emotional labor also speaks to how jobs that require being "nicer than natural" and good at handling people, such as is the case with waiters, waitresses, receptionists, flight attendants, and nurses, can force individuals to suppress their true feelings when carrying out their tasks. To the extent that technology and emotional labor divorce individuals from feelings in general, they could distort perceptions about how comfortable others are discussing a particular topic. (As a reminder to the reader, contrary to what the latter point might suggest, the focus in this chapter is not on the emotional aspect of caritas, which will be addressed in the next chapter, but on its discursive dimension.)

WHAT MAY BE BEHIND THE VEIL OF PLURALISTIC IGNORANCE THAT PREVENTS NURSES' SPIRITUAL TALK

Applied to nurses, these literatures would suggest that nurses' spiritual talk is subject to misperceptions and second-guessing depending on three conditions—the *prominence of an issue* (whether a subject is often an item for discussion at official meetings), *interpersonal networks* (whether work units are large and impersonal or small and intimate), and *sociotechnical conditions* (whether work requires considerable energy focusing on the functioning of equipment and the acting out of emotions). What is less clear is whether these factors shape perceptions separately or jointly. Being in a work unit where a particular issue is prominent, for example, might be enough to enable one to accurately perceive others' opinions about it regardless of one's interpersonal networks and sociotechnical conditions. Or the prominence of an issue may be consequential depending on one's location in social networks and/or the sociotechnical nature of one's tasks.

Therefore, it is important to test two possibilities. The first is that the prominence of an issue, interpersonal networks, and sociotechnical conditions all matter independently: each one affects pluralistic ignorance in its own way. The second is that different combinations of these factors produce different causal pathways to pluralistic ignorance. Whether these conditions act independently or jointly will determine exactly how pluralistic ignorance prevents nurses from discussing spirituality and, therefore, prevents caritas as a language from flourishing in clinical settings.

METHODS

Data

I examine these two possibilities using data drawn from a real-life example of pluralistic ignorance where group members (nurses) gathered at the same physical site (University Hospital) tend to misperceive one another's feelings about discussing an ultimate concern (spirituality). Very few studies have collected data on actual instances of pluralistic ignorance among assembled peers. The standard practice has been to describe alleged cases of pluralistic ignorance (e.g., students not asking questions in class) and then speculate about their causes (cf. Prentice and Miller 1993). To the extent that empirical analyses are conducted at all, they are typically done under laboratory or computer-generated conditions. The data used here are also unique in that they allow us to explore different manifestations of pluralistic ignorance—that is, why some group members who embrace a minority opinion falsely impute their opinion to the majority and some in the majority falsely impute their opinion to a minority.

In addition to their relevance to caritas, I focus on hospital nurses and their talk about spirituality for two other reasons. First, some researchers claim that nurses are the type of group that is prone to pluralistic ignorance (Miller and McFarland 1991). According to them, pluralistic ignorance occurs under conditions that facilitate the mutual observability of group members, heighten the salience of group identity, and pressure members to present a public facade of professionalism. All three conditions apply to hospital nurses. Second, spirituality is the type of ultimate concern that Eliasoph and Lichterman (2003) suggest is often subject to an unpopular speech norm. That is, it is a topic that many individuals are privately interested in and would like to discuss but often do not because they are under the false impression that most of their peers are uncomfortable with it. In part, this is because the groups to which they belong focus on more doable projects (e.g., treating the observable, physical symptoms of a patient) and therefore avoid discussing problems viewed as more difficult (e.g., addressing the invisible, transcendent worth of the sick).

Measures

I assess the presence of pluralistic ignorance among nurses by comparing their answers to two questions about conversations within their work environment. The first asks nurses how strongly they agree or disagree with the statement "I am comfortable talking about spirituality." The second asks nurses how strongly they agree or disagree with the statement "Most coworkers (fellow nurses) are comfortable talking about spirituality." Answers to both items are coded 1 = Strongly Disagree, 2 = Disagree, 3 = Agree, and 4 = Strongly Disagree.

While spirituality can be communicated in a variety of subtle ways (e.g., by wearing sacred jewelry) and can take on rather frivolous meanings, when nurses refer to "talking about spirituality," they usually have in mind explicit conversations about matters of deep, existential significance. For instance, when asked in an open-ended survey question to describe an event that had a significant (positive or negative) impact on their understanding of spirituality, all of the 210 (of 299) nurses who answered this question described incidents involving dying or suffering individuals. Likewise, when a group of 20 nurses was asked in postsurvey interview sessions what they had in mind when they answered the survey question about whether other nurses are uncomfortable talking about spirituality, all but two referred to talk about incidents of dying or suffering. Therefore, when respondents answered the survey question about whether their coworkers are comfortable discussing spirituality, they were not referring to how they think their coworkers will fill out a survey but what they perceived in their daily interactions with them. Finally, consistent with the holistic philosophy of care promoted at the hospital studied, all of the nurses in postsurvey interviews said they were aware that spirituality can be expressed using somewhat different vocabularies (e.g., biblical versus New Age).

Qualitative researchers are correct to note that there are limits to studying meanings like spirituality in a strict survey format (Bender 2003). These sorts of limitations are not unique to our study. When other researchers have analyzed the pluralistic ignorance surrounding, for example, racial attitudes, they have typically relied on survey data (e.g., Greeley and Sheatsley 1971). Their reason for doing so is obvious: surveys provide an estimate of a group's majority opinion and individuals' perceptions of that opinion. This information, in turn, can be used to test the relationship between perceptions and hypothesized causal factors.

Therefore, while our closed-ended survey questions do not allow us to explore a host of issues about spiritual talk that might be interesting, they do allow us to determine, in a way not possible with only descriptive methods, whether a statistical majority of nurses feels comfortable or not talking about spirituality, which nurses misperceive this normative opinion, and which factors have nontrivial relationships with these misperceptions. As the reader will see, I did, though, elicit qualitative comments about whether spiritual talk took place among coworkers in interviews with nurses, which gave me further insight into what nurses felt about the absence or presence of such conversations.

With respect to our key predictors of pluralistic ignorance, I gauge the prominence of an issue using a survey item that asks whether spirituality frequently comes up at staff meetings and briefing sessions. Interpersonal network is captured using two indicators—a variable that indicates whether or not a nurse works in a hospital unit with an above-average number of registered nurses and a survey question about whether or not nurses think that their job offers chances to make friends with coworkers. Sociotechnical conditions are measured using two variables. One asks nurses whether they agree or disagree with the statement "My work is largely dictated by technology." The other is a two-item measure of emotional labor that asks nurses whether they agree or disagree with the statements "I often feel I cannot be myself at work" and "I often have to fake how I really feel at work."

In the appendix to chapter 4, I discuss these predictors in more detail. There I also discuss the statistical techniques used to determine how the three sets of predictors independently and jointly shape how nurses perceive their coworkers' ease about discussing spirituality.

THE DETERMINANTS OF PLURALISTIC IGNORANCE AMONG NURSES

Preliminary Findings

Before this study's survey was fielded, the head of the hospital's Nursing Division was asked whether she thought it is easy for the nursing staff to discuss matters of spirituality. She answered, "I think it is fairly easy for them. I am making my assumption based on the fact that they have chosen to work here in a hospital. And those things are tied in with the service we provide. So, I think they would be comfortable with it." In contrast, research on pluralistic ignorance would suggest that group members may still not talk about topics like spirituality if they misperceive that most of their peers are uncomfortable engaging in such conversations. Consistent with this argument, survey results revealed that while an overwhelming majority of nurses (85 percent) said that they themselves are "comfortable talking about spirituality," only a minority (43 percent) believed that their coworkers (fellow nurses) are. The latter discrepancy is a clear example of pluralistic ignorance.

As table 4.1 indicates, when we look more closely at the 173 (of 299) respondents who incorrectly perceived the majority opinion, we find that 44 of these nurses were uncomfortable talking about spirituality *and* 38 of them believed that most other nurses are uncomfortable with such talk. We label this group the "incorrect minority." On the other hand, 135 of the 173 were comfortable talking about spirituality *and* believed that most other nurses are uncomfortable. We label this group the "incorrect majority."

Figure 4.1 shows that in most nursing units, well over 50 percent of nurses said they are comfortable discussing spirituality but falsely

TABLE 4.1

Accuracy of nurses' attributions of majority and minority opinions

	I am comfortable talking about spirituality	I am uncomfortable talking about spirituality	
Most coworkers are comfortable talking about spirituality	120 (40%)	6 (2%)	126 (43%)
	Correct majority[a]	Correct minority[b]	
Most coworkers are uncomfortable talking about spirituality	135 (45%)	38 (13%)	173 (57%)
	Incorrect majority[c]	Incorrect minority[d]	
	255 (85%)	44 (15%)	299

[a] Nurses in the majority who correctly impute their feelings about spiritual talk to most other nurses.
[b] Nurses in the minority who correctly impute their feelings about spiritual talk to a minority of nurses.
[c] Nurses in the majority who incorrectly impute their feelings about spiritual talk to a minority of nurses.
[d] Nurses in the minority who incorrectly impute their feelings about spiritual talk to most other nurses.

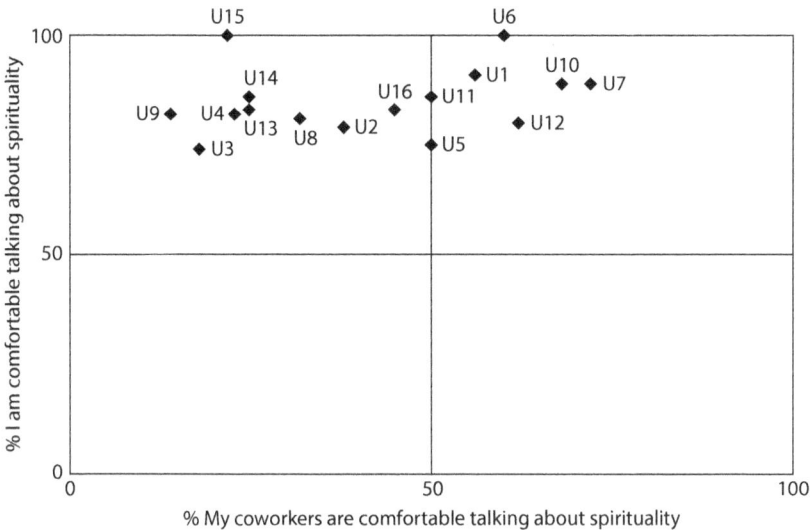

FIGURE 4.1. Variations in pluralistic ignorance across hospital units.

perceived that fewer than 50 percent of their coworkers are comfortable. This tendency to misperceive the majority opinion was particularly great in major units like the operating room and the emergency department. In contrast, in five units, well over 50 percent of nurses said they are comfortable discussing spirituality and correctly perceived that more than 50 percent of their coworkers are as well. Nurses in the pediatric intensive care unit, for instance, had especially accurate perceptions. The fact that the accuracy of nurses' perceptions varied so greatly across these units suggests that the silence surrounding spirituality cannot be attributed just to a taboo against discussing such topics. Instead, it likely has to do with conditions that shape the visibility of others' opinions.

Independent Determinants of Misperceptions

To ascertain what factors might cause nurses to misperceive how comfortable their coworkers are discussing spirituality, a statistical analysis was conducted that assessed the independent effects of our key predictors. This analysis also took into account whether respondents themselves are uncomfortable talking about spirituality. Findings reported in figure 4.2 show that *the prominence of an issue* exerts a significant effect on misperceptions; that is, nurses who attend meetings where spirituality is frequently discussed are much less likely to be guilty of pluralistic ignorance. Their odds of misperceiving the majority opinion about spiritual talk are 0.339 of those who attend meetings where spirituality is not often discussed. The size and potential intimacy of a nurse's *interpersonal network* also significantly influence pluralistic ignorance. Specifically, nurses' odds of misperceiving the majority opinion are increased by 1.554 if they are in a unit with an above-average number of coworkers. And the odds that nurses will misperceive their coworkers' feelings about spiritual talk are reduced by nearly 0.329 if their work context lends itself to making friends, as is often the case in units requiring extensive teamwork. Finally, results indicate that pluralistic ignorance is a function of *sociotechnical conditions*. The odds that nurses will misperceive the majority view increase by 1.417 and 1.610, respectively, if their work is dictated by technology and requires the suppression of feelings, as is the case in units like the operating room and emergency department. These findings support the possibility that each key predictor has an important net impact.

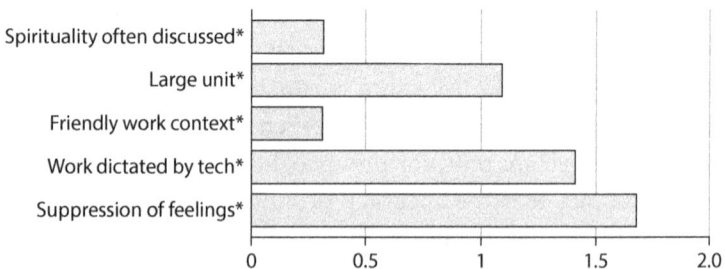

FIGURE 4.2. The odds that nurses will misperceive coworkers' comfort about spiritual talk.

The Conjoint Determinants of Misperceptions

However, it still might be the case that some of these predictors work in concert, which would be in keeping with our second prediction, which suggests that the factors that shape the visibility of others' opinions could interact in complex ways such that the effect of one factor may be contingent on the presence or absence of the others. To find out whether and how these factors work together, I conducted another analysis that tested whether our key predictors combine to produce different empirical pathways to pluralistic ignorance. Here I used a statistical procedure that can identify the minimal set of configurations needed to cause nurses to misperceive the majority opinion. These pathways are defined in table 4.2 by factors that are present (indicated by filled circles) and those that are absent (indicated by empty circles).

Results revealed that there are two distinct combinations or pathways associated with pluralistic ignorance. Interestingly, one of these pathways

TABLE 4.2
Pathways to misperceiving other nurses' comfort about spiritual talk

	Pathway 1	Pathway 2
Prominence of an issue		
Spirituality is often discussed at official meetings	○	○
Interpersonal networks		
Larger-than-average unit size		●
My job offers chances to make friends with coworkers		○
Sociotechnical conditions		
Work is dictated by technology		●
Work requires suppression of feelings	●	●
I am uncomfortable talking about spirituality	●	○
Odds ratio	7.221	6.461

● Condition present

○ Condition absent

describes the conditions that produce the "incorrect minority" effect, while the other describes the conditions that produce the "incorrect majority" effect. To be more precise, the minority of nurses who are uncomfortable discussing spirituality are prone to misperceive the majority opinion if they are in a unit where spirituality is rarely discussed at official meetings *and* they experience an above-average level of suppressed feelings or emotional labor. Their odds of misperceiving the majority opinion are 7.221. The majority of nurses who are comfortable discussing spirituality tend to misperceive the majority's view where spirituality is rarely discussed at official meetings, in units that are above average in size, in jobs that do not provide opportunities to make friends with coworkers, in jobs dictated by technology, *and* if they experience an above-average level of emotional labor that requires the suppression of feelings. For this latter group of nurses, then, the pathway to pluralistic ignorance is more complex, suggesting that for those who are comfortable talking about spirituality, several more conditions need to be in place for them to be persuaded that their coworkers feel otherwise. Their odds of misperceiving the majority opinions are 6.461.

To determine the robustness of these pathways, I analyzed their effects alongside those of other potentially relevant factors. Even when I controlled for these other influences, the two pathways or configurations both have a significant impact on whether nurses misperceive their peers' feelings about discussing spirituality. This finding further supports the possibility that pluralistic ignorance is the result of different combinations of visibility factors. It also suggests that the barriers to invoking caritas as a language in clinical settings cannot be reduced to any single factor. Rather, they are created by complex sets of conditions that lead frontline care workers to misperceive their coworkers' feelings about spiritual talk.

Discussion

This begs the question: where within a hospital are the two identified pathways to pluralistic ignorance most like to develop? We can answer that question by identifying nurses who possess or lack these pathways' combinations of attributes. For example, suppose one wanted to gain more insight into the "incorrect majority" pathway and how it relates to some of the units depicted in figure 4.1. We can do this by examining the nurses that have all or none of the conditions associated with this effect. Consistent with what was observed in figure 4.1, most of the nurses with all of these conditions are from the operating room (U3), whereas all of the nurses having none of these conditions are from the pediatric intensive care unit (U7). This finding points to the locations where within University Hospital the "incorrect majority" effect is most and least likely to occur.

Specifically, it indicates, on the one hand, that the conditions that cause nurses who are comfortable talking about spirituality to misperceive that most other nurses are uncomfortable are especially likely to be present in the operating room. There, the topic of spirituality is not likely to come up or be prominent because of the lack of regular nurse-patient interactions. Most patients are unconscious when brought to the operating room and remain so during their entire stay there. Operating room nurses also have less interaction with a patient's friends or family members because the latter are not permitted in the operating room. Because operating room nurses have few opportunities to learn about the spiritual anxieties of their patients and their companions, it follows that they also have less information on these matters to report at staff meetings and briefing sessions.

In addition, the operating room has the second largest nursing staff (seventy-three) in the hospital, which makes canvassing the unit's majority opinion more difficult than in smaller units. Operating room nurses must employ highly sophisticated tools (e.g., electrosurgical equipment) according to detailed protocols and under the direct watch of their superiors (surgeons). These technical and social pressures, in turn, may render nurses less sensitive to spiritual sentiments and hinder the formation of deep, transparent friendships with their peers. And in the operating room, where work is focused almost exclusively on the physical state of patients and dealing with crisis situations in an efficient manner, emotional displays by nurses may be less tolerated or considered out of place, making it more difficult to discern any feelings that coworkers might have about spirituality.

On the other hand, nurses from the pediatric intensive care unit (PICU) have few if any of these conditions. Unlike their counterparts in the operating room, they must regularly interact with severely ill children and their anxious guardians. Deep, existential issues, therefore, have a much greater chance of surfacing at the bedside and being discussed at official group gatherings. Indeed, other survey results indicate that nearly a third

(30 percent) of nurses in the PICU report that spirituality comes up frequently in staff meetings and briefing sessions, compared to only 2 percent of operating room nurses. (That there is not unanimous agreement in the PICU that spirituality is often discussed at official gatherings is likely due to the fact that different nurses work different shifts that can change from week to week.) While it would be great to observe these meetings and learn exactly what was said about spirituality in them, our survey at least allows us to pinpoint where within hospitals spirituality is most likely a regular item on meeting agendas.

In addition, the PICU has a smaller nursing staff (twenty-one), which makes the discernment of the majority opinion easier. The size of this unit, combined with the fact that its nurses often work in the absence of physicians, also facilitates the development of intimate friendships among peers. Nurses in the operating room and the PICU both use highly sophisticated tools. However, because PICU nurses are primarily responsible for the minute-by-minute care of their patients, they exercise more discretion in the timely application and adjustment of technology. PICU nurses are also more involved in ethical decisions about the continued use of lifesaving equipment. This may partly explain why half (50 percent) of operating room nurses say that their work is largely dictated by technology, whereas a much smaller percentage (15 percent) of PICU nurses express this opinion. The fact that all patients in the PICU are children, who are generally considered blameless for their physical ailments, also creates an emotionally charged work setting where nurses' outward displays of grief, anger, and other emotions are more accepted.

CONCLUSION

It can be hard to introduce spiritual talk into secular settings, and that includes nurses in public hospitals. One reason it's hard is pluralistic ignorance: people misjudge how common their own opinions are among their peers. Among nurses, some contextual factors make it easier and harder for nurses to accurately gauge their colleagues' interest in talking about spirituality and spiritual care: the prominence of an issue, interpersonal networks, and sociotechnical conditions play important roles in making others' feelings about the subject transparent. These factors are also likely to converge at particular locations within a hospital, such as the operating and emergency rooms, and be absent in others like the pediatric intensive care unit.

Results thus challenge the conventional wisdom that people refrain from invoking the language of spirituality because it might offend others. People may perceive that others would be offended, but that perception can be wrong. In the case of nurses, most welcome talking about spirituality, and in that sense caritas as a discursive phenomenon has create potential to stick. But nurses' feelings about the topic are cloaked by other factors, creating an atmosphere ripe for second-guessing.

This finding brings to mind an essay by William James titled "On a Certain Blindness in Human Beings," in which he describes the challenges of being aware of another person's inner life. James draws on a story by Robert Louis Stevenson about a group of young boys who create a secret club of "lantern bearers" who hide small tin lanterns under their heavy winter coats as a sign of membership. Observed from the outside, they look like anyone else scurrying through the cold night. But when they meet, they lift the edge of their coats to reveal a hot burning light hanging from a belt loop. Similarly, as people who address human affliction, many nurses share an interest in the spiritual dimensions of personhood but are often unaware of belonging to the same "club."

One consequence of this pluralistic ignorance is that nurses' spiritual lives are largely mysteries to their fellow nurses. In the words of one charge nurse, "I know one nurse in labor and delivery who doesn't really believe in God at all. Yet, she's nevertheless a very supportive and healing kind of person. So, there's some inner strength there that she's getting but I do not how she is getting it." Similarly, when asked in a presurvey interview what question about spirituality he would pose to workers in his unit, a nurse answered, "I would just like to know how many people are thinking about this stuff [spirituality]. Does it cross their minds? You have all of these evangelists on TV and so forth. Do they think like them? . . . I really don't know." Or, as another nurse more succinctly put it, "I would like to know what fills my colleagues' tanks." (We will examine some of nurses' rarely shared thoughts and experiences in a later chapter.)

To shed more light on this outcome and others like it, we need to better understand the strategies that individuals use to engage and discern issues that matter to their peers (see Bender 2003). For example, when asked what might determine whether nurses talk about spirituality, some nurses suggested that a nonjudgmental attitude can open up conversations about it. According to one of them, "What I notice is that very few people are willing to volunteer a lot if they think you are critical. If they believe you to be sympathetic, it's a lot easier for them." The same nurse also suggested that humor, when used with caution, can be a means to get others to talk at a deeper level. "When a patient says something like 'If the Lord is willing,' I will sometimes reply, 'Maybe He's not so willing today.' I just tease and that sort of thing because people do better with humor. They don't seem to feel like there's so much mortal danger if the people around them are a little less serious. . . . But you have to be careful. A lot of people make money these days poking fun at religion [and] that can be offensive to some." Another nurse spoke of how she will sometimes deliberately annoy coworkers to find out where they stand on the issue of spirituality. "Sometimes I'll fish. I'm very curious about people . . . And so, I will occasionally stir the pot, seeing if people will get emotional. I've been accused of being an antagonist . . . If you want to measure the people around you, get them emotionally involved in a conversation about religion."

In some instances, nurses discovered by accident that spirituality mattered to others, as occurred in this incident with a patient:

> I had a patient who was on an artificial heart device and he was called to transplant one night. We got him all ready, and he went through the surgery, but died as soon as he got to the ICU. What comforted me during this time was the ecstatic expression he had on his face as they were wheeling him to the O.R. . . . I cherished all of the funny things he used to say and do. But I also remembered two occasions when I found him in his room next to his bed, kneeling on the floor. I asked him what he was doing. I thought maybe he had fallen—but he wasn't hurt. He said "nothing" and looked embarrassed. Looking back on it now, my coworkers and I think he may have been praying.

Presumably, had this nurse been given more time to get to know her patient, it would have been less difficult for her to make sense of his actions.

Results suggest that hospitals might take some practical steps to address the factors that hinder spiritual dialogue among staff, which, in turn, could help legitimate the practice of spiritual care in clinics. When comparing the two pathways to misperceptions shown in table 4.2, we notice that two conditions are shared by each—emotional labor and discussions of spirituality at official meetings. Focusing on these visibility factors might, therefore, be a good starting point for addressing the second-guessing surrounding spirituality. We will address the issue of emotional labor in the next chapter, as well as how nurses' ability to express their true emotions is facilitated or inhibited by the promotion of spirituality in hospitals. Here we simply note several strategies used in the past by workers to minimize the negative effects of emotional labor, such as recognizing the pressures at hospitals to compartmentalize feelings, commending colleagues who manage their feelings well in the face of challenges, making sure that the burden of suppressing feelings is only asked of a select set of workers skilled at regulating their emotions, and providing flexible arrangements to vent anger or other emotions. To the extent that these strategies enable nurses to be more open about feelings that are evoked by exposure to human suffering, they could help make the concerns that anguish also raises about spiritual matters easier to share.

With respect to discussing the spirituality of official meetings, short of forcing the topic to be a regular agenda item, units could occasionally make time to remind nurses of spirituality's likely place in their work. For example, one could inform nurses and their peers that they probably share an unspoken interest in spirituality because of their constant exposure to human suffering, just as teachers must sometimes tell their students who hesitate to raise their hands that their classmates probably have similar questions about a subject. Hospital administrators might also encourage staff to make more time to talk about what they fear others consider to be "stupid questions," including those of a spiritual nature that surface when dealing with matters of life and death that staff members may perceive are only of interest to them. And frontline staff might be advised to develop the habit of identifying situations in which they assume they feel one way and others feel another way and to ask themselves whether they might be misunderstanding what others are experiencing. Of course, it is imperative that hospitals provide the resources needed to make such adjustments. Otherwise, they could simply place an additional burden on nurses.

By the same token, staff should be encouraged to discuss whether spiritual talk is necessary at all. Some might welcome such talk and benefit from it, others may view it as intrusion and a threat to their work and well-being, and still others may consider it unwarranted, as in the case of the operating room, where spiritual care could be important to nurses but their patients are unconscious. Regardless of where staff members stand on the issue, by making it an open topic of conversation, they should be in a better position to move beyond unspoken speech rules that give rise to pluralistic ignorance to more explicit ones that foster mutual understanding.

Staff may also discover that even when they share the same religious background, they can still misperceive one another's spiritual thoughts, as I did my dad's just before our transplant procedure. This experience further sensitized me to how misperceptions surrounding spiritual talk might prevent caritas from being integrated into modern life.

On Sunday, the day of my dad's surgery, he and I take a walk from the Family House to downtown Pittsburgh, where worship services at several of its historic churches are ending. All are towering stone edifices, some of which are open for afternoon tours. According to a plaque on its black iron fence, Trinity Cathedral is the "oldest unreconstructed landmark" in the city. It rests on a former American Indian burial ground deeded by William Penn's heirs to the congregation's forefathers. A little over one hundred marked graves of an estimated four thousand people buried there still remain, including Dr. Nathaniel Bedford, Pittsburgh's first physician and a founder of the University of Pittsburgh. Inside Trinity, tourists find hand-carved pews of white mahogany and a stone pulpit with intricate carvings of prophets, saints, and bishops. Some of the stained-glass windows date back to 1872.

Not far from this cathedral is First Presbyterian Church, which features thirteen 26-foot by 7-foot stained-glass windows designed by Tiffany Studios, each costing over $3,000 when the church was opened in 1905. Inside the narthex are two 80-foot ceiling beams and a pair of rolling, two-ton, 30-foot oak doors leading to the sanctuary, where one can find carved birds, animals, and insects on its interior stonework as well as an eagle, butterfly, and dove on the pulpit. Also nearby is Smithfield United Church of Christ, whose 80-foot aluminum steeple was the first to be made of such material in the world. Inside its sanctuary is a 19-foot rose window made in 1860 and twelve soaring, stained-glass windows displaying scenes from the Bible and Pittsburgh's history, including an 1861 visit by President-elect Abraham Lincoln.

While touring these historic churches and gazing on their teeming and creative expressions of the divine, I reflect on how much of the religious past has been erased by the sanitized present. Few might be aware that the University of Pittsburgh Medical Center (UPMC) Montefiore Hospital, where our transplantation is to take place, has its roots in Judaism. It was founded in 1908 by the Ladies Hospital Aid Society as a place where Jewish physicians were welcome to practice, Jewish patients could be cared for with dignity and understanding, and the achievements of Jewish health care could be shared with patients of all faiths and races. Just as it is hard for me to imagine that a section of liver could be taken from one individual and regrown in another, I suspect it is equally difficult for some to fathom that Montefiore Hospital stemmed from these religious sources.

As we walk through Pittsburgh's historic churches, I realize that these and related thoughts are probably of little interest to my dad, who is losing touch with reality. He is enveloped in a mental fog caused by the ammonia seeping to his brain, a condition that will only worsen until the transplant. I think we might ground him temporarily if we go a few blocks northeast of downtown to a church of his own denomination— First United Methodist Church of Pittsburgh. It was founded in 1946 as part of a merger between the German-speaking Evangelical Church and the United Brethren in Christ. It is an equally impressive building with a gray-tan stone facade and iron roofs covered with red Akron tile. When we arrive, we discover that it does not have any scheduled tours. Instead, it is conducting an outdoor "blessing of the animals" service.

Liver patients act differently when ammonia permeates their brains. Some become extremely confused and anxious, while others are drowsy and disoriented. In my dad's case, ammonia occasionally causes him to become mischievous. Unbeknownst to me, he has slipped into the latter mode as we walk by the animal blessing service.

He insists that we wait until the service ends so that he can ask the presiding pastor a question. Given that he is just hours away from a life-and-death procedure, I presume it is about something of deep concern that he would only feel comfortable discussing with a fellow pastor. Instead, when the service concludes, he approaches the pastor, tightly grasps his hand, and asks, "Reverend, do you think my doggie is going to hell?" He spins away giggling with his hand over his mouth. His ploy reminds me of a lesson I'd learned years earlier as a chaplain: never second-guess the spiritual impulses of others.

Chapter Five

PATHWAYS TO SPIRITUAL MEANING AND EMOTIONAL DEAD ENDS

If caritas is to stick in modern public life, it's not enough for helping professionals to think that their otherwise mundane tasks of caregiving can be spiritually meaningful. The factors that enable them to view their work in a spiritual light must also contribute to their emotional well-being. Indeed, there's considerable suspicion about inserting spiritual understandings into scientized care settings because they may be used to exploit workers' feelings. After all, science was developed in part to rid the world of manipulative forms of magical thinking that had previously robbed people of their agency—their personal power and ability to affect their own lives. I knew that religion could be emotionally exploitive before I entered the chaplaincy program, but I became acutely interested in this issue after an encounter with a chaplain intern.

During the interpersonal relations seminar (IRS), which was held in a second-floor conference room, Clinical Pastoral Education (CPE) chaplain interns and part-time students were asked to discuss some of the tensions they experienced between their personal lives and their professional roles as chaplains. Some commented on how difficult it was to emotionally detach themselves from certain patients, especially children in the pediatric intensive care unit, and to deal with their passing. Others wondered aloud if they were cut out for this work and how much they really had to offer patients, noting that they often received more strength from patients' courageous examples than vice versa. The IRS also functioned as a backstage where we could joke about our clumsy interactions with certain patients and staff. Stories were told, for example, of trying to pray with a patient who continually passed gas, what an x-ray might reveal of another with a bad temperament, the patient who claimed he had a type of allergy for which there was no cure—white people—and what would happen if the chaplain intern who was skeptical of miracles was assigned to all patients who watched the 700 Club and expected to be divinely cured.

At the same time the IRS facilitated poignant and comical exchanges, it occasionally degenerated into an amateurish exercise of scrutinizing the feelings of one's peers. This was especially likely when interns and students were asked by the CPE director to comment on one another's clinical experiences. For example, one might speculate that an intern cut a patient visit in the oncology unit short because he or she had yet to come to grips with the death of a relative or his or her own mortality. Or someone who visited an above-average number of patients—a rate buster of sorts—might be accused of being controlling or seeking others' attention.

In my case, the chaplain intern who hoped to develop a harp ministry in hospice settings expressed concern that my academic training was preventing me from getting in touch with my true feelings and was imposing a professional facade between patients and myself. She noted that being "authentic" and willing to be transparent was not just a requirement of a Rogerian approach to therapy. It was also what made our work as chaplains spiritual.

From the time I declined to partake of an addition to her aroma therapy kit that she passed around at one IRS session, she continually reminded me of my seeming reluctance to connect with patients and emote in their presence. In one sense, she was on to something: displaying feelings was a learning process for me and something that I did sparingly for fear of intruding into patients' lives. Still, her accusations felt harsh and misplaced, both to me and to some others in our group. Once she went so far as to declare, "Don, I think you really need to work on getting out of your head." The oldest chaplain intern responded, "Instead of asking others to get out of their heads, why don't you work on prying your head from your harp."

I did not participate in their ensuing argument, but it did lead me afterwards to reflect on the issue of authenticity and the harp chaplain's claim that our work was "spiritual." She was echoing the director, who had taught us that embracing our work as spiritual care would enable us and our patients to be more emotionally real. While the harp chaplain apparently bought into that idea without question, I didn't know the director well enough to take his word for it. Indeed, it struck me that to do as he instructed and simply believe that chaplaincy was spiritual would have been like caving in to the pressure of an altar call, leaving me feeling manipulated. I had to discover for myself whether this type of work was truly spiritual. For the first weeks in the program, I was not sure. I did not sense that patients really needed my help. But after a seriously ill patient confided in me about her fear of death and sharing that experience with the oldest chaplain, I became convinced that there was something spiritual about my role.

The irony, though, was that those types of patient situations and my clumsy responses to them also sometimes made me wonder if I was simply putting on an act. I was expected to project calm and assurance when sometimes I really felt inadequate to the task and unable to imagine what it would be like to suddenly learn, as these patients had, that one's life had taken a grave turn. This made me realize that perhaps it was not so much believing that one's work was spiritual that engendered feelings of authenticity or inauthenticity as the circumstances that led one to that belief. Tending to extremely sick patients, for example, might convince one that one's care was spiritually important, but it could also pressure one to fake or suppress one's emotions when performing one's role, especially when there was nothing in one's training that addressed how to deal with such pressures.

As Weber noted, rationalization is impersonal. And today, in the highly rationalized setting of a research hospital, care professionals often say that they long for a more humane, personal work environment in which they can genuinely relate to their clients. According to one physician in University Hospital's integrative medicine program, "I talk, we all talk about the importance of being real, of being authentic. Being with a patient, you know, when we sit with them in the clinic. And it makes a huge difference. . . . People really appreciate the authenticity, the ability to listen to them, to be caring. They pick up on that. And for me, it's really powerful." Partly in response to this yearning for authenticity, this doctor's hospital and several others like it have sought to emotionally liberate staff by promoting humanistic meanings like spirituality that, according to their religious and nonreligious advocates, speak to the inherent goodness of individuals.

But, as I discovered in my exchange with the harp chaplain, spiritual responsibility sometimes comes with emotional expectations that can feel excessive. As a chaplain intern, I felt pressured to display more feelings than came naturally to me. Others at University Hospital made a related observation that some workers who view their work in spiritual terms seem emotionally worse off. According to the staff chaplain, "There are lots of nurses here who have a heart for caring for people and it goes beyond the letter of the job description. They are the ones who really try to relate to patients as whole persons, as beings with a soul. They do the best job of caring for people. But they are also sometimes the ones who pay the highest emotional price."

So, which is it? Does believing their science-based work has spiritual significance make caregiving emotionally rewarding for nurses? Or might it be detrimental to their emotional well-being, exacerbating negative states like feeling phony?

One way to address this issue would be simply to compare the feelings of nurses who do and do not describe their work in spiritual terms. If nurses who believed their work was spiritual were more likely to say they felt inauthentic, then one could conclude that internalizing a spiritual understanding of care tends to be emotionally harmful and vice versa. But, as I learned in my experience as chaplain, the issue is more complicated than that, and such comparisons do not begin to address why nurses feel the way they do. What can make a corporate-sponsored meaning emotionally beneficial or harmful is the particular pathway an individual takes to adopting it.

The question addressed in this chapter, therefore, is: why might nurses believe their care is spiritually significant, and how does that belief shape whether they feel more or less authentic at work? As it turns out, sociologists have long been interested in the emotional well-being of workers and how employers will occasionally try to shape their feelings by promoting certain company values. Reviewing this literature provides clues about the conditions under which nurses at University Hospital might come to think of their work as spiritual and how those conditions, in turn, can shape their feelings of authenticity. Consistent with this body of work, I find that nurses take different routes to adopting the spiritual understanding of care promoted by their hospital but that only some of these routes also engender positive feelings of authenticity.

This fact suggests that for caritas to emotionally resonate with care workers, it is not enough for corporate leaders to just tell them that their work has spiritual import. Other experiences at work and elsewhere will decide whether they internalize that interpretation. And should few of the pathways leading them to see their work as spiritual generate feelings of authenticity, the survival of caritas will have to depend more heavily on other mechanisms identified by Weber to transmit this religious ethic.

SEEKING DEEPER INSIGHT INTO THE EMOTIONAL CONSEQUENCES OF ADOPTING CORPORATE-SPONSORED SPIRITUAL MEANINGS

Emotions at Work

The subject of "emotions at work" has been a central concern for sociology since its founding. Durkheim (1997) observed that as societies modernize, they increasingly divide labor up by specializing into distinct occupational groups. He argued that this division of labor can foster positive feelings of belonging and solidarity among people in the same line of work. Marx (1867) challenged this view, claiming that capitalism exploits the working class, engendering negative feelings of anger and alienation among wage earners. Weber (1958c), in turn, predicted that rationalization would reduce laborers to "cogs in a machine" and drain employment of meaning, causing human feelings (both positive and negative) to disappear from work.

Interest in the subject continued into the twentieth century, when scholars began to question Weber's thesis that the modern workplace is antithetical to meaning and emotional displays. They observed that businesses frequently use mission statements, orientation workshops, training manuals, and other normative devices to instill workers with company values (Kunda 1992). In the process, businesses also induce employees to exhibit certain feelings, a feature of work life that Hochschild (1983) has labeled "emotional labor."

Contemporary scholars disagree, though, over the implications of these tactics for workers' psychological well-being. Critical scholars stress how corporate efforts to "engineer values" and ensure that "service is delivered with a smile" bend workers' emotions into unchosen and unnatural shapes (Kunda 1992; Hochschild 1983, 2003). Others suggest that normative techniques can enhance workers' emotional health if they are not used solely to improve productivity. These scholars, who align with notions of bounded emotionality, compassion at work, or moralized markets, argue that companies can optimize their effectiveness *and* make work a more authentic experience by promoting meanings that resonate with workers' deeper sensibilities (Mumby and Putnam 1992; Zelizer 2017).

Recent debates in health care over the field of nursing illustrate these issues. Many argue that hospitals have struggled to attract and retain nurses, despite improvements in their pay, because modern medicine focuses on diseases rather than sick persons. Thus these paid caregivers are discouraged from relating to patients on an intimate, human level and often become disillusioned with their jobs. Optimistic reformers argue that hospital management can effectively treat patients and free nurses to express heartfelt concern for them by promoting more holistic under-standings of care. By this, they do not mean that hospitals should aban don biomedical technologies and replace them with largely unproven therapies advocated by the holistic medicine movement. Rather, they mean that hospitals should adopt an approach to health that cares for individuals' physical and nonphysical needs, including their spiritual ones. According to optimists, this approach would improve patient sat-isfaction as well as make caregiving a more meaningful and authentic experience for nurses. Critical scholars (Hochschild 1983; Reich 2014; Gordon 2007) argue the opposite—that holistic ideologies exploit nurses' spiritual impulses and further reduce them to "prisoners of compassion." From their perspective, attempts to imbue caregiving with spiritual meaning would alienate rather than authenticate nurses in the same way portraying nurses as selfless angels demeans their occupation's status as a scientific profession.

Weber could not have anticipated employers' recent attempts to infuse the workplace with meaning and the controversies this effort would spark among academics about its emotional consequences. However, in arguing that meaning arises through a process of interaction, he did suggest that corporate-sanctioned meanings cannot simply be imposed on workers. Rather, whether employees adopt the understandings espoused by their employers will likely depend on intervening factors that influence how employees make sense of those understandings. This insight has important implications for whether caritas "lands" in nurses' emotions because the particular pathway that a worker takes to a corporate-sanctioned meaning may produce feelings of authenticity or inauthenticity.

As we will see in a later section, proponents of a negotiated order perspective have developed Weber's point further, suggesting the various ways that meanings can be created and maintained within organizations (Hughes 1958; Strauss et al. 1963; Becker et al. 1976; Fine 1984; Hallett 2003). According to this framework, the heads of major corporations cannot create organizational cultures, instrumental or expressive, by fiat (cf. Peters and Waterman 1982). Instead, whether employees adopt a corporate-sanctioned meaning, and with what emotional effect, depends on the conjunction of several social conditions: employees' relationships with supervisors, clients, and one another; their preexisting interpretive frames; and their involvement in outside institutions. Organizational cultures, in other words, are defined by the different conditional pathways to meaning and the different emotions attached to those pathways.

Before turning to the negotiated order framework, it is important to review why Weber's prediction that work would be drained of meaning and emotion did not materialize. This helps us better understand how believing their care is spiritually significant can make nurses' work more emotionally rewarding or more emotionally burdensome.

Weber's Fear About Work Becoming an Iron Cage

The history of American business did not fully bear out Weber's fear that rationalization would lead to a meaningless and emotionless "iron cage" (Gouldner 1954; DiMaggio and Powell 1983). While many owners initially sought a bureaucratic and technical solution to the problem of management (Braverman 1974), protests from labor (especially during the contentious 1920s and 1940s) forced them to rethink how to manage employees and their emotions. Companies and their consultants developed a human relations (HR) model of management (Mayo 1945; Maslow 1998) that sought to improve morale and strengthen company loyalty by making work more intrinsically rewarding.

Managers tried to ease the burden of wage work by offering various material amenities that they believed would address workers' social needs. For example, Ford established its famous "five-dollar day" program that paid workers a certain share of company profits if they met efficiency standards and ran their homes in a similarly disciplined fashion. But managers also used "softer" strategies, such as workplace rituals to stimulate a feeling of community and new framings of the company as a unitary corporate "team" (Whyte 1956). With the emergence of the service economy and new forms of information work, many of these classic HR strategies have been revived and refined, with workers encouraged to relate to their customers and their jobs on a deep, emotional level (Kunda 1992; Kunda and van Maanen 1999).

Softer forms of control have always generated controversy among those who worry that they will emotionally burden employees (Leidner 1993). As Hochschild (1983) famously described, employers may demand that workers engage in "deep acting": conscious strategies to manipulate not only their emotional displays, but their inner emotional states as well. However, workers bring to their tasks other expectations of themselves that they use in evaluating whether their work behavior is consistent with their true selves. Hence, when companies assign meanings to work that are not in accord with employees' system of values, they create within workers a disjuncture between the self-as-presented and the self-as-experienced (Goffman 1956; Erickson 1995; see also Taylor 1989). The need to be authentic or behave in a manner that is consistent with one's values (Erickson 1995) is especially acute among knowledge and care workers. Because they place more weight on the intrinsic rewards of work, such as a sense of fulfillment and emotional satisfaction (Kelley 1985), their sense of authenticity and commitment to a firm depend in part on the opportunities they are given to express their self-values.

Increasingly, firms attempt to link workers' "authentic" self-understandings with the needs of the organizations—to the supposed benefit of both. Rather than dictating exact "feeling rules" for workers to follow, employers today encourage employees to put their own passions to work on assignments. Managers often use the prospect of more authentic work to justify corporate restructuring and other cost-saving measures (Kunda 1992; Barley and Kunda 2004; Boltanski and Chiapello 2005). They claim, for example, that by shedding expensive bureaucracies, companies can free frontline service workers to pour their "hearts and souls" into client interactions. Especially in industries facing chronic shortages of skilled, professional workers (such as nurses and software developers), managers have felt it necessary to use strategies that imbue work with deeper meanings.[1]

Unless companies provide these coveted free agents work that enables them to express their deepest values, they risk losing them in an economy that increasingly favors mobile workers. While the health care industry has been part of his development, it has not gone as far as the corporate Silicon Valley types that provide laundry and ping pong on site or We Work locations adorned with throw pillows imploring tenants to "Do what you love." Rather, it has sought to give caregivers permission to relate to patients on a deeper, human level. Some scholars also hold out hope that the expressive needs of workers can be balanced with the instrumental ones of business (Mumby and Putnam 1992). While acknowledging that there are limits to the meanings that can be derived from certain tasks, they contend that companies can still integrate workers' deeper needs with those of the organization.[2]

One important—and perhaps unintended—consequence of these developments has been the reinsertion of "spirituality" into the workplace. As Bell and Taylor explain (2003), some managers and business consultants now encourage employees to appreciate the spiritual significance of their work and even to view it as a calling. This notion of work as a calling was common in the United States in its early days; according to Weber, Protestantism encouraged people to work hard as a spiritual duty, and wealth earned through hard work was seen as a sign of salvation. Now, secular managerial ideology is curiously reviving this sacred work ethic—this time not as a way of demonstrating one's status among the "saved," but as a way to work more meaningfully within capitalism. As one nurse explained, "I think part of the reason I really enjoy being a nurse is that it is part of a larger calling. . . . People who approach their work spiritually can handle patient care better. A lot of people let this work and its frustrations get to them. That's why spirituality has a lot to do with being able to handle this work." This comment speaks to the strength that spirituality provides this nurse. At the same time, it suggests the huge emotional burden that can be placed on individuals if they are made solely responsible for spiritual care. She makes no mention of her institution's responsibility to equip nurses to deal with the emotional challenges that spiritual care might create.

Academic medical centers like University Hospital have recently sought to fill a chronic shortage of nurses, in part, by portraying the profession in more holistic terms, as one that allows compassionate individuals to express their concern for others' bodily and spiritual needs. In their recruitment campaigns, for example, hospital administrators often advertise nursing as work fit for "angels of mercy." In doing so, they are trying to affirm more intimate understandings of care that many think have been betrayed by modern hospitals that stress detached concern over emotional expression. They suggest further that in giving nurses permission to believe that their care has both physical and spiritual import, hospitals can improve the satisfaction of patients who complain that biomedicine ignores their existential concerns (see McGuire 1993; Bone 2002).

Critics, however, question whether more humane forms of care are possible in modern hospitals, given their increasing reliance on advanced technology and the ongoing rationalization of medicine (see Erickson and Grove 2008). Nor do they trust that hospitals will reward the special skill and emotional effort that go into providing spiritual care (Gordon 2007). They suspect that hospitals are really trying to commodify caregivers' innermost values. In advertising their commitment to providing holistic care, hospitals may also prime patients' spiritual expectations in ways that nurses are not emotionally prepared to meet (see also Ashforth and Vaidyanath 2002). For example, nurses may feel pressured to affirm patients' sacred identities while still having to subject them to "profane" procedures like physical exams that threaten to strip those identities away (Goffman 1961).

So, will spiritual care take hold emotionally for nurses and other care workers? The verdict is out. If companies are responsive to caregivers' understandings, as optimists suggest, then the answer may depend on whether individual caregivers already hold spiritual beliefs that might align with a spiritual understanding of their work. But if incorporating spirituality can be a form of commodification and alienation, as critical scholars suggest, then the answer may depend on caregivers' work environments.[3] Rather than studying the impact of individual and environmental factors separately, this chapter explores how they might work together. It asks: Are nurses more likely to internalize a spiritual understanding of their work under some working conditions than others? How do these different conditions, in turn, shape nurses' feelings of authenticity or inauthenticity? Answers to these questions can help us understand some of the conditions that might make caritas emotionally sustainable.

HOSPITAL CULTURES AS NEGOTIATED ORDERS

The negotiated order perspective is particularly helpful in addressing the question of how corporate spirituality might affect workers emotionally because it offers a conceptual model that deals explicitly with meanings and the factors that lead individuals to adopt work-related understandings. Proponents of the negotiated order perspective were the first scholars to use the phrase "organizational culture," and their work has made it clear that rationalization is altering the experience of "sentimental work," especially in hospital settings (Hughes 1958; Strauss et al. 1963; Becker et al. 1976; Fine 1984). The negotiated order perspective also differs from managerial theories that suggest that leaders can conspire to change work cultures to their liking. It argues instead that the meanings of work espoused by leaders are subject to negotiation. That is, for workers to accept company-sanctioned understandings, those understandings must resonate with workers' interactions with colleagues and clients, previously acquired cognitive frames (the mental templates that individuals use to make sense of the world), and their experiences in other institutions.

In a nutshell, the negotiated order framework rejects the notion that rationalization empties work organizations of meaning and emotion. It also rejects the idea that there exist prefabricated cultures that executives can simply select and impose on workers. In this framework, work cultures develop as workers take multiple, interactive pathways to adopting the meanings their workplace promotes, and these different pathways are associated with different feelings about those sanctioned meanings.

The next section discusses in more detail the four sets of conditions identified by negotiated order scholars that may render organizationally sanctioned meanings like spirituality more or less plausible in the minds of coworkers: vertical work relations, horizontal work relations, cognitive frames, and involvement in outside institutions.

Dimensions of Work Culture

VERTICAL RELATIONS

Negotiated order scholars suggest that organizational cultures are shaped by the vertical relations between staff and superiors (Strauss et al. 1963; Hallett 2003). While administrators are well positioned to define work situations, they cannot force their definitions on workers. Instead, they must convince subordinates that administrators' definitions are plausible and relevant to their work contexts. Especially when dealing with knowledge workers and other core personnel, they must act less like authoritarian chiefs and more like confidantes if they are to persuade employees that their understandings of work are valid. As companies like hospitals continue to eliminate middle layers of management, responsibility for transmitting corporate understandings and gaining workers' trust increasingly falls upon frontline supervisors (see also Boltanski and Chiapello 2005). For example, when asked about the positions, besides those of chaplains, that would be eliminated at University Hospital due to budget shortfalls, the perinatal unit's supervisor commented, "It will mean more projects for supervisors in the areas of education, human resource development, etc. . . . We are hoping bedside workers who were not cut, like nurses, will feel comfortable asking us questions about the changes, that they feel there are open lines of communication." This statement speaks to the challenges that frontline supervisors face in the wake of downsizing in trying to gain the trust of subordinates.

HORIZONTAL RELATIONS

Even if supervisors can win the confidence of workers, the latter may still be unwilling to embrace corporate-sanctioned meanings. Acceptance of those meanings is also contingent on workers' horizontal relations with peers and clients (Strauss et al. 1963; Hallett 2003). With respect to peers, relationships within an occupational subculture at work can strongly influence an individual's response to managerial ideology (see Lively and Heise 2004; Lively 2006). Such relationships may be especially important when it comes to adopting unconventional understandings of work. Nurses might be more inclined to believe that their highly rationalized work also has spiritual significance, for example, if they have coworkers who embody that meaning through their deep concern for one another (see Berger and Luckmann 1966). In fact, some at University Hospital went so far as to describe their coworkers in familial terms, such as this nurse: "I have great coworkers . . . We are really a team and the girls are like my little sisters, my big sisters . . . It is nice to be loved as a person and as a friend by the females. And the guys, they are great . . . Some days we have a blast. We go out as a group a lot of times, it's kind of fun. Extremely rewarding."

With respect to clients, employees' receptivity to more intimate meanings of work may be influenced by the extent to which they are involved in "sentimental work" that requires them to relate to clients as "alive, sentient, and reacting" beings (Strauss et al. 1982).[4] Members of caring professions like nursing perform such work, although it varies depending on their social skills, the technical nature of their duties, and the seriousness of their clients' situation (Chambliss 1996). That is, some nurses may feel more adept than others at gaining patients' confidence. Some may have to treat patients using equipment that is frightening or painful and thus create existential dilemmas. And nurses who work with patients who are chronically ill or have terminal conditions may be more involved in intimate aspects of the self. These dimensions of sentimental work may, in turn, condition whether nurses can view their tasks in spiritually meaningful terms, since they determine nurses' exposure to existential issues often raised by human suffering.

COGNITIVE FRAMES

Other negotiated order research suggests that the plausibility of a meaning may depend less on interaction than on individuals' preexisting cognitive frames or interpretive schemes. Snow and Machalek (1982) argue that unconventional ideas about the end times, past lives, the efficacy of prayer, and other issues persist in the face of disconfirming evidence partly because most individuals do not think in deductive, scientific terms. That is, they do not always evaluate others' claims according to their internal consistency or ask what kinds of empirical events are needed to disprove them.

Instead of using analytic, scientific logic, many people approach spirituality using synthetic logic; that is, they interpret reality based on their experience of it. Synthetic logic may be more conducive to a sense of spiritual meaning than analytic logic is. So it may be easier for nurses and other workers to find their technical tasks deeply meaningful if they don't rely on scientific logic as a test of validity and instead draw conclusions based on personal experience.[5] They may assume that things normally considered dualities (e.g., mind/body, personal/technical) are really interconnected, but without specifying the nature of those connections and the type of evidence needed to disconfirm them. One of the chaplain interns described such a mindset:

> For me, spirituality is the connectedness with people, the oneness of God, the oneness of the universal energy that we all share. You know how some people fill you with energy and other people zap you of energy? When I look at the whole area of spirituality, I don't view it as some esoteric thing. Rather I look at it more as physical reality . . . when you connect with a patient's heart, you can actually feel the neurological energy . . . you have a closeness to them unlike anything else . . . and so when people die they are actually feeling themselves transcend into the next stage of the journey . . . energy cannot dissipate when we die.

While some might dismiss this type of thinking as a sign of cognitive weakness, its synthetic logic may allow for a more expansive moral imagination than a purely scientific one.

INVOLVEMENT IN OUTSIDE INSTITUTIONS

No company exists in a vacuum; companies are always nested in a larger field of competing organizations. So when a company promotes a particular meaning or value, such as spirituality, it's doing so amid other organizations that sometimes claim ownership of the same cultural meaning (Hallett and Ventresca 2006). Traditionally, it was churches and other religious organizations that most closely associated themselves with spirituality. The fact that some secular hospitals are now sanctioning spirituality suggests that churches and other religious organizations may be losing their traditional monopoly on spirituality and the sacred (see Bellah et al. 1985).

Such interinstitutional competition creates a situation where workers may embrace the same corporate-sponsored meaning but for different reasons. To stay with the example of hospitals and spirituality, some nurses may believe that their work has spiritual import because their participation in religious communities sensitizes them to the sacredness of life. Slightly more than a fourth (29.4 percent) of the nurses examined here attended religious services on a weekly basis, and over a third (37.7 percent) at least monthly. Conversely, some nurses' aversion to religious institutions may prompt them to view work (as opposed to churches) as a primary outlet of spiritual expression. As noted in chapter 3, a quarter of the nurses at University Hospital agreed or strongly agreed with the statement "I feel more spiritual at work than elsewhere." Given that church participation has diminished over the past few decades to where less than half of Americans are members (Jones 2021), this finding would suggest that even if involvement in religious communities does lead individuals to embrace spiritual understandings of their work, a smaller and smaller number of workers in the future will follow this path.

RECAP AND PREDICTIONS

To sum up what has been said so far, nurses, like other helping and knowledge professionals, place a premium on authenticity, defined here as behaving in ways that are congruent with one's values (Erickson 1995). To retain these vital employees, corporate leaders often tell them that corporate restructuring and other cost-saving measures create new opportunities to realize their values and, therefore, they should begin thinking of their tasks as an expression of those values. In the case of nurses, hospital administrators have tried to justify streamlining operations by suggesting that this streamlining will free nurses to relate to patients on a more personal level, allowing them to believe that their otherwise technical work has deep, spiritual significance.

Scholars have also debated the implications of these corporate strategies for care workers' emotional well-being. Optimists contend that organizations are being responsive to care workers' values, suggesting that workers who already belong to outside institutions that support spiritual beliefs will embrace their employer's promotion of spirituality and benefit from it emotionally. Pessimists argue that in endorsing spiritual understandings, organizations are trying to manipulate care workers' yearning for authenticity. They suggest that if such meanings take hold, it will likely be due to more mundane conditions at work that effectively pressure workers to adopt corporate-sponsored spirituality, further alienating them from their true feelings.

Negotiated order researchers suggest that while management is in a unique position to define situations, subordinates possess substantial flexibility in how they perceive their work environment. Hence, these scholars would expect that horizontal relations at work, cognitive framing, and involvement in outside institutions would each have a direct bearing on whether workers adopt a meaning promoted by their corporation.

By the same token, these researchers suggest that there is no single, optimal configuration of conditions that leads workers to adopt a meaning. Instead, there may be a variety of pathways that lead different workers to adopt a corporate-sponsored meaning (Fiss 2007). If that's true, then workers' emotions may also depend on the particular pathway they take to a meaning.

The Possible Pathways to Spiritual Meaning and Their Implications for Nurses' Feelings of Authenticity

Applied to the study at hand, these arguments translate into three predictions:

1. Hospital administrators just telling nurses that their care has spiritual import doesn't automatically mean that nurses will believe it. Rather than being shaped by vertical relations at work, nurses' adoption of this interpretation will be directly influenced by their horizontal work relations, cognitive framing, and involvement in outside institutions.
2. Nurses' adoption of this meaning may also be conditioned by how these factors interact.
3. Depending on the interactive pathway they take, nurses' sense of authenticity at work will likely vary. And of these pathways, the ones most likely to engender positive feelings of authenticity are those involving participation in religious institutions.

METHODS

I tested these predictions using a survey item that asked nurses how strongly they agreed or disagreed with the statement "There is something spiritual about the care I provide." I assessed how dimensions of their work culture influenced their answer to this question using nurses' responses to questions about their vertical and horizontal work relationships, cognitive frames, and involvement with religious institutions. And I appraised nurses' feelings of authenticity using a two-item scale that measured how strongly nurses agreed or disagreed with the following statements: "I often feel I cannot be myself at work" and "I often have to fake how I really feel at work." The appendix to chapter 5 provides additional information on the variables and statistical methods I used to test these predictions.

Obviously, how emotions are managed by care organizations varies (Lopez 2006). At one extreme are highly coercive organizations that dictate how employees are to feel when enacting a corporately sanctioned understanding of care. At the other extreme are those that do not prescribe feeling states but provide resources for negotiating and developing caring relationships. The hospital studied here leans toward the latter. This and the fact that it operates largely on public funds suggest that feelings of inauthenticity may be less common in this hospital than in a more top-down, profit-oriented organization.

Some might object that, for this reason, it would be more appropriate to investigate workplace emotions in more private, cutthroat businesses than in a public or university-affiliated hospital. However, it is important to point out that the logic of the market, of profit making, increasingly pervades all health care organizations via new institutional templates such as the HMO and managed care (Starr 1982). Hospitals, even public and university-affiliated ones, are more likely today to be run by administrators with degrees from business schools than by health care specialists (Scott et al. 2000). In this respect, the profession of nursing looks increasingly like any other form of wage labor under capitalism, making University Hospital's nursing staff an important case study to see how meanings promoted by organizations to legitimate the rationalization of operations shape workers' emotions (see Gordon 2007).

WHY NURSES ADOPT A SPIRITUAL UNDERSTANDING OF THEIR WORK AND ITS EMOTIONAL CONSEQUENCES

Preliminary Findings

Prior to administering this study's survey to nurses, the head of the Nursing Division was asked if she thought most nurses considered spirituality to be a part of their work. "I don't think anyone would be resistant to spirituality . . . I would like to believe that by virtue of the profession they have chosen or the field they are working in, it is the kind of compassion and care you would show somebody . . . I have come across people who believe, you know, that prayer is pooh-pooh and all those things, that they were not convinced those sorts of things work. But I have to say I have never come across a nurse who objected to spirituality." While she stopped short of saying whether nurses actually found their work to be spiritual, survey results indicate that most do. In the hospital examined here, 86 percent of the nurses strongly agreed or agreed with the statement "There is something spiritual about the care I provide."[6]

The Direct Effects of Work Culture

Figure 5.1 provides insights into what factors convince nurses that there is something spiritual about the care they provide. It summarizes the results of an analysis of the direct, independent effects of vertical relations, horizontal relations, cognitive frames, and involvement in outside institutions on the strength of this belief. Conditions that exert a statistically significant impact on nurses' belief that there is something spiritual about their care are indicated with an asterisk. The strength of these conditions' effects is captured by the horizontal bars that represent each factor's standardized coefficient.

Consistent with the idea that workers need to trust supervisors if they are to adopt corporate-sanctioned meanings, this figure reveals that nurses are more apt to believe that their care has spiritual significance if they can confide in a supervisor about spiritual matters ("Trusts supervisors"). However, as the figure also shows, this indicator of vertical relations also falls short of being statistically significant. With respect to horizontal

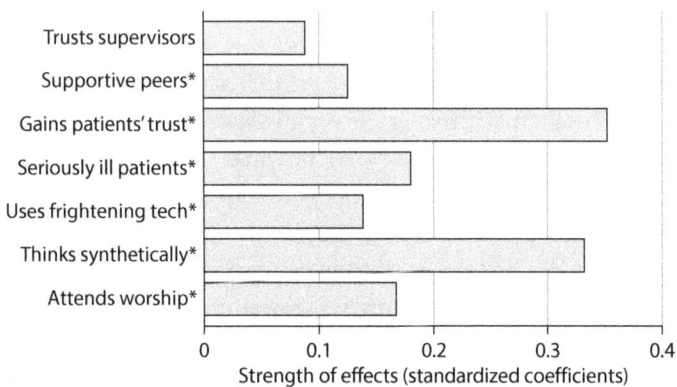

*Statistically significant

FIGURE 5.1. Determinants of nurses' agreement with the statement "There is something spiritual about the care I provide."

relations, findings show that all four measures have a significant influence on workers' beliefs. Specifically, nurses find the spiritual import of their tasks more plausible when they feel supported by their coworkers, think they are competent in gaining patients' trust, treat patients with serious conditions, and use technology that elicits negative reactions like fear from patients, which can add to the existential concerns raised by suffering. In terms of cognitive frames, to the extent that nurses interpret reality according to a synthetic logic, they are more inclined to believe that their mundane tasks have spiritual significance. Conversely, this would suggest that employing a strict, scientific logic inhibits nurses' ability to view their work in such a light. Finally, nurses who regularly attend worship services are more likely to interpret their acts of care in a spiritual light. In general, findings reported in figure 5.1 support the prediction that horizontal relations, cognitive frames, and involvement in outside institutions shape workers' adoption of corporate-sanctioned meanings. Of these factors, being able to gain patients' trust and thinking synthetically are the most associated with this outcome.

The Combined Effects of Work Culture

Another statistical analysis was carried out to determine whether the prediction that these conditions act synergistically or combine to determine the same outcome holds true.[7] The results are summarized in table 5.1, which shows the different pathways to nurses' spiritual understanding of care. These pathways are defined by factors that are present (indicated by filled circles) and/or those that are absent (indicated by empty circles).

Findings reveals that there are five pathways to the belief that "there is something spiritual about the care I provide." None of these pathways, however, is shaped by the trustworthiness of supervisors.[8] Instead, they are influenced by the other three sets of conditions—vertical relations, cognitive frames, and involvement in outside institutions.

Specifically, nurses who take the first pathway consider themselves skilled at gaining patients' trust, work with patients who have serious conditions, use technology that is not frightening to patients, and think synthetically. Nurses who take the second consider themselves skilled at gaining patients' trust, work with patients who have serious conditions, think synthetically, and regularly attend worship services. Nurses who take the third have

TABLE 5.1
Pathways to spiritual understanding of care and their consequences

	Pathway 1	Pathway 2	Pathway 3	Pathway 4	Pathway 5
Vertical relations					
Trusts supervisors					
Horizontal relations					
Has supportive peers			●	●	●
Gains patients' trust	●	●	●		●
Has seriously ill patients	●	●		○	●
Uses frightening technology	○		●	○	○
Cognitive frames					
Thinks synthetically	●	●	●	●	
Involvement in outside institutions					
Attends worship		●		○	○
"My work is a calling"	YES	YES	YES	NO	NO
Emotional outcome	Inconsequential	Authenticating	Inconsequential	Alienating	Alienating

● Condition present

○ Condition absent

supportive peers, consider themselves skilled at gaining patients' trust, use technology that is frightening to patients, and think synthetically. Nurses who take the fourth have supportive peers, work with patients who do not have serious conditions, use technology that is not frightening to patients, think synthetically, and do not regularly attend religious services. Finally, nurses who take the fifth pathway have supportive peers, consider themselves skilled at gaining patients' trust, work with patients who have serious conditions, use technology that is not frightening to patients, and do not regularly attend religious services.

I also analyzed whether other potentially relevant factors, such as age and years of education, might explain the significance of these five pathways' relationships to nurses' beliefs about the spiritual significance of their care.[9] In every instance, these pathways still had a statistically significant effect on whether nurses believe that their care is spiritually important, when factoring in these other potentially relevant variables.[10] Hence, results support the prediction that a worker's adoption of a corporate-sanctioned meaning is influenced by how nurses' horizontal relations, cognitive schemes, and involvement in external institutions interact. This finding suggests that spiritual understandings of care can be transmitted to the level where care is actually delivered through not one but multiple routes.

Another analysis was also conducted to determine whether the five pathways listed in table 5.1 influence a similar outcome—whether nurses consider their work a "calling."[11] In our sample, 23 percent of nurses believed their work to be a calling, compared to 60 percent who considered it a career and 17 percent who thought of it as a job. The results of this analysis are summarized in the lower panel of table 5.1 (see "My work is a calling"). It reveals that three of the five pathways have positive and statistically significant associations with the calling measure. While these findings indicate that the two outcomes are not one and the same, they also suggest that they are influenced by some of the same combinations of factors.[12]

Different Pathways to Meaning Have Different Emotional Consequences

So, what are the emotional consequences of these different routes to meaning? Do some of them seem to lead more to positive feelings than others? We next investigate the extent to which the five configurational pathways just identified also lead to feelings of authenticity. For the sample as a whole, fairly small percentages of nurses reported that they often fake their emotions. Specifically, 10 percent strongly agreed or agreed with the statement "I often feel I cannot be myself at work," and 14 percent strongly agreed or agreed with the statement "I often have to fake how I really feel at work."[13] Also, when these two indicators of inauthentic feelings are combined into a scale, there is an insignificant correlation between it and the key outcome, belief that there is something spiritual about one's care ($r = -0.050$). However, rather than concluding that belief in spiritual care is irrelevant to feelings of inauthenticity among these nurses, it may be that the relationship between the two depends on the pathway a nurse takes to that belief.

As we see in the lower panel of table 5.1 (see Emotional outcome), this turns out to be the case.[14] Nurses who take the first and third pathways adopt their hospital's spiritual understanding of care with a negligible impact on their self-feelings. Their type of spiritualism can be characterized as *emotionally inconsequential*. Nurses who take the fourth and fifth pathways adopt the same spiritual interpretation of care but suffer from emotional dissonance. Theirs is an *emotionally alienating* spiritualism. And nurses who take the second pathway adopt their hospital's spiritual rendering of care and experience emotional consonance. Theirs is an *emotionally authenticating* type of spiritualism. This pathway requires nurses to be skilled at gaining patients' trust, to work with seriously ill patients, to think synthetically, and to attend worship services regularly. Importantly, this pathway is also the only one that involves participation in religious institutions. Results, then, are consistent with the prediction that nurses' feelings of authenticity will vary depending on the route that they take to a corporate-sanctioned meaning, and of these, only the route that includes a commitment to organized religion makes nurses feel authentic.

CONCLUSION

With reference to the problem of how caritas could survive in highly scientized, public settings, one possible solution might be to have those who supervise helping professionals to promote and thus legitimate spiritual understandings of care. Several corporate leaders, in fact, have come to think of their role in such terms, as indicated by the titles of best-selling books like *Leading with Soul* (Bolman and Deal 2011). But, as results presented here show, administrators' ability to impart spiritual values pales in comparison to the influences of colleagues, patients, mindsets, and outside institutions. These conditions directly and conjointly shape whether nurses can view their tasks in spiritual terms. Moreover, not all of these conditions that make the spiritual plausible allow care workers to feel they are being true to themselves. Of the five conditional pathways uncovered here, only one enhanced nurses' sense of being authentic. Interestingly, this was also the lone pathway that involved attendance at worship services, which has dropped off precipitously in recent years ("State of the Church 2020" 2020), suggesting that this route has become even more narrow over time.

In short, findings show why it is naive to assume that workers will follow the ideological lead of management or adopt corporate-sponsored meanings for the same reasons. They also cast doubt on the argument that workers are mere "carriers" of institutions and therefore are ready to take up whatever meanings their organizations espouse (Creed, Scully, and Austin 2002).[15] Most importantly, they suggest that while it may still be possible for the spiritual meanings associated with caritas to stick in modern hospitals, many, if not most, of the avenues leading to such understandings are emotional dead ends. This situation is exacerbated by the fact that hospitals like the one examined here give nurses few resources to understand and cope with the extra emotional weight that spiritual care may put on them. While this is obviously not ideal for the survival of caritas, it's not necessarily a death knell either. In the next two chapters, I consider why caritas might still endure despite the emotional sacrifice it seems to require.

Still, not even nurses who throw their hearts and souls into their work can wholly make up for the alienation patients experience. Emotions and spirituality can recede into the horizon as patients experience their bodies being swiftly prepared and stationed for surgery in environments that are designed to save lives but not to promote feelings of safety and comfort. This was my experience at the transplant center.

It's a humid, rainy night when a cab pulls up to take my dad and me from the Family House to the transplant center. Our family will follow us and make the same trip an hour later, just before the procedure begins at midnight, which the surgical team thought was necessary because of my dad's rapidly worsening condition. The driver seems to have traveled this route before, because when we tell him our destination, he wishes us both well and even tries to comfort us by telling us about other patients he knows of who had successful operations. At first I wonder whether he may be a hospital employee who's been told to reassure passengers, but I see on the license posted on his dashboard that he's an independent contractor.

The large waiting area is empty except for a janitor who is gathering his mop and sponges in a bucket and preparing to wheel them away. In contrast to the outside darkness, the room's overhead lamp and orange, faux leather couches are strikingly bright. Sitting there and listening to the rain against the high windows feels like hanging out at a lonely diner.

When two nurses finally arrive, they take us to separate hospital wings. I am escorted to a small room where I change into a hospital gown and slip-resistant socks. I am then led to the end of a long corridor, where I am to wait in a semiprivate room for the next two hours. A curtain separates me from the other patient until he moves it aside and introduces himself as Doug. Doug lives in Pittsburgh and worked for a while at one of its famous steel-making furnaces before it closed in the early 1980s, after which he took a job as a high school janitor. Doug is waiting for his second cadaveric liver transplantation in three years.

After sharing where I am from and why my dad and I are here, I lie back on my bed staring at the squares of acoustical ceiling tile. I am hoping to reflect and calm myself before being taken to the next station. But Doug apparently finds the ensuing silence awkward and peppers me with questions at five- and ten-minute intervals. In particular, Doug wants to know if I have physically prepared myself for the procedure and understand just how painful it is. I tell him that during the preceding weeks I had gone through a conditioning program designed by a long-distance coach, but Doug is unconvinced that it will be enough.

Doug explains that because narcotics linger in the bloodstream longer than other meds and your new or (in my case) regenerating liver may not efficiently process pain killers like morphine at first, patients must endure excruciating pain shortly after they awake. Getting yourself in good cardio shape may help you endure and survive the procedure, Doug exclaims, but immediately afterwards nothing can really help you. NOTHING. The pain is so deep and intense that you wish you would DIE. I suspect that Doug is a bit of a drama king, but his excessive openness is unsettling all the same, and I feel anxiety welling up. I try cutting the discussion short by diverting his attention and asking how Doug prepared himself for his second procedure. Proudly patting his beer belly, he grins and responds, "Obviously, not with a cardio routine."

Eventually I escape Doug and am transported from our room to another section of the hospital, where I am prepared for surgery. It is a cold, almost frigid room whose darkness seems to stretch in every direction but the floor. It has the cavernous feel of an abandoned warehouse with walls and ceilings too distant to touch and see. Like the dim hallways that I roamed during my nights shifts as a chaplain, it seems to absorb sound and emotion from the air. The rubber tires of the medical stretcher that carry me in are barely audible, and then go completely silent when I am parked and left alone under a low-hanging lamp.

I hear faint footsteps coming toward me. Two faces suddenly appear from out of the dark and directly over me, encased by the lamplight's glow. A bespeckled, middle-aged man puts an anesthesia mask over my face and asks me to deeply inhale. To his right a nurse with shiny black curls and a thick Russian accent discusses with him where I am to be taken upon falling asleep. I study her eyes for signs of assurance. She eventually reaches over to rub my brow and says, "We will take care of you and your dad."

She, the light, and the air around me soon melt into shadows.

Chapter Six

STYLES OF SPIRITUAL CARE

I wanted to know not only what convinces nurses that their care is spiritual and whether that makes them feel authentic, but also when and how they put spiritual understandings into practice. After all, the core meaning of caritas is actively nurturing vulnerable strangers as spiritual beings. I first became interested in this issue when I realized that chaplains' "care" can hurt people if they're not careful. One chaplain intern, for example, shared during a Clinical Pastoral Education (CPE) case seminar how he upset a dying patient by offering to say a prayer, only to be told by the patient that she had been rejected by her church because she was a lesbian. I wondered more about how to enact caritas as my chaplaincy internship continued and discovered that I was only rarely called upon for help. But the importance of skilled action really came home to me on one occasion when I was called on for my services and found that my fledgling chaplain's toolkit was painfully inadequate.

One of the purposes of the CPE case seminars was to better understand what patient encounters revealed about our relational style. It also provided the CPE director with an opportunity to identify practices that were deemed unhelpful and might tarnish the reputation of his program. He told us that in previous years some chaplain interns had taken it upon themselves to prescribe fixes to patients' spiritual problems; the most egregious example was an intern who had told a cancer patient that he must recite certain Bible passages before receiving chemotherapy. Others had made the mistake of offering prayer to individuals who had been ostracized by organized religion, as one of the interns in our group confessed to.

Requests for explicitly religious therapies, in fact, were rare. During my six months on the night shift, for example, only eight people asked for prayer (a man who learned that his cancer was inoperable, a parent whose young daughter needed a heart transplant, a couple whose child was about to be put on life support, a mother whose two daughters had been killed in her auto accident, a father whose son with Down syndrome was dying, a family of fifty who had been misled to believe their grandfather's cancer had been cured, a mother whose newborn was about to undergo exploratory surgery, and a guilt-ridden man who had been told by family that he was sick because did not attend church), three asked for baptism (one in the neonatal intensive care unit and two in labor and delivery), two asked for communion (both in the cardiovascular intensive care unit), and one asked for a Bible (in ambulatory surgery).

Still, well-meaning chaplain interns could sometimes abuse such therapies or apply them when they were not wanted. To solve this problem, the director promoted a particular intervention that seemed the least capable of doing harm: reflective listening. This approach was perhaps best summed up in a framed quote by John Wayne in the conference room—"Talk low, talk slow, and don't say too much." Being somewhat of an introvert, I felt comfortable with this less intrusive technique and the Rogerian framework upon which it was built, which stressed empathizing without getting personally involved in others' problems. It also comported with the habits that had been drilled in me as a social scientist that emphasized the importance of maintaining a professional distance. And yet I occasionally wondered about its appropriateness in settings like hospitals where the reality of human suffering was undeniable. Was it really enough to restate or reflect back what patients say, for example, about their fear of death? I doubted it, but I was not given any other therapeutic training. I worried as well whether I was attracted to reflective listening because it absolved me of any wrongdoing in much the same way that people feel a lack of accountability when following bureaucratic rules.

Whatever my doubts about the approach and its effectiveness, my fellow interns and the director felt that I had what they considered a "breakthrough" as a Rogerian practitioner during my sixth month in the program. It was at the end of a night shift, when I was paged to meet in the emergency room with a couple whose toddler had just been declared dead from a pool drowning. The mother was beside herself with anger and screaming at her husband, whom she blamed for her daughter's death. The father eventually ran out of the small waiting room, leaving me alone with the mother.

Before I had a chance to introduce myself, a nurse brought in the deceased child and put her in the seated mother's arms so that she might say "goodbye." The mother held the child closely and cried uncontrollably. I was at a total loss as to what I should do. The primary intervention I had been taught as a chaplain, reflective listening, felt utterly useless and out of place. So, I decided to just to be there with her, and my presence did seem to calm her some. As my shift neared its end, I bent over and put my business card on the chair next to her, inviting her to contact me if she felt another visit would be helpful. But as I rose, I caught a glimpse of her child. She was roughly the age of our firstborn. The serenity of her face and the beauty of her delicate lashes startled me, as they reminded me of our daughter lying asleep. I suddenly knelt next to the mother, speechless.

The chaplain intern who came to replace me reported to others that I seemed to be crying. I didn't remember crying, but my peers, including the harpist, took my alleged tears as evidence that I had achieved a new level of empathy and transparency, and they never told me I needed to open up again. As far as I was concerned, though, the event proved nothing—except perhaps that academics like me kiss our kids goodnight like most everyone else.

But that incident also prompted me to think about what practices other staff members, and especially bedside nurses, use when dealing with patients who are experiencing spiritual stress. What arrows did they have in their quiver, and under what circumstances did they employ them?

When people enter a hospital, they often experience a degrading shift from person to patient. The small, thoughtful gestures of loved ones that validate their intrinsic worth and infuse everyday life with meaning disappear just when they're needed most: when people are betrayed by their own bodies or, in the case of the mother whose infant drowned, when a loved one is tragically stolen from them. In the words of a chaplain intern, "The hospital is sort of like a dark desert. People are stripped of what's familiar, stripped of their clothing, stripped of control of their lives, and must work to make sense of it all with little clue as to what lies ahead."

Hospital workers are surrounded by people facing uncertain futures. But they may feel, as I did, that there are few opportunities to provide spiritual care. As one nurse explained,

> When I went to nursing school, instructors put a lot of stress on patients' emotional and spiritual needs. We did a lot of role-playing on how we would deal with certain situations. But I think we all knew that in the real world we weren't going to have much time to do that. I mean, we learned things like massage and helping patients who might be in pain, we learned to distract them using imagery techniques and so forth. But, from my experience, I really do not have a lot of time on the floor to do that.

A significant percentage (46 percent) of nurses at University Hospital shared that view, answering that they disagreed or strongly disagreed with the statement "My work provides many opportunities to put spirituality into practice."[1] Workers may also feel that when such opportunities do arise, the interventions they have been taught seem ill suited to the situation, as I did with reflective listening when asked to console the grieving mother. Whatever the case may be, knowing when and how to show spiritual sensitivity can be challenging in the "dark desert" of hospitals.

This dilemma was foreshadowed in Weber's (1978) essays on social action. Weber was deeply interested in the meanings people attribute to behavior. He believed that people choose their actions based on their social context and what kinds of actions are considered meaningful within that context. Scientific settings, he argued, severely constrain the range of meanings that workers can impute to their interactions: practical, technical, and impersonal meanings are highlighted, while spiritual, moral, and personal meanings are seen as illegitimate. The result, Weber argued, is that workers are reduced to "specialists without spirit." Scientific hospitals require nurses to focus on impersonal protocols and technical procedures—those are the actions that are considered legitimate and meaningful in that context. But caritas requires moral actions that dignify strangers as spiritually important human beings. What's it like, then, to try to add caritas into such a technical environment? Weber feared that this combination would be extremely difficult for paid care providers to pull off.

Whereas Weber described this moral quandary in broad, conceptual terms, Erving Goffman (1956) later detailed how it manifests itself among mental health workers in his famous study on total institutions, organizations where people are cut off from the wider community and placed under formal control. He wrote: "It is important therefore to see that the self is in part a ceremonial thing, a sacred object which must be treated with ritual care. We are thus led to the special dilemma of the hospital worker . . . his occupational role obliges him to care . . . in a place of unholy acts and unholy understandings, yet some of them retain allegiance to the ceremonial order outside the hospital setting." In other words, care workers, on one hand, are responsible for enforcing bureaucratic rules and applying scientific methods that effectively rob patients of their identities and replace them with others that are oriented to the authority and smooth operation of institutions. Upon entering an emergency room, for example, patients are required to change into a hospital gown and instructed that family and friends must leave or step aside as trained staff perform a thorough physical exam. On the other hand, workers are obliged to create an environment that dignifies vulnerable strangers, one that treats them less like physical objects and more like spiritual subjects by engaging in acts that affirm their sacredness as humans. How workers respond to this dilemma, according to Goffman, likely differs depending on their commitment to reproducing the wider society's rituals for respecting and honoring others. These rituals range from practices promoted by churches such as praying for the sick to less explicitly religious ones like holding a patient's hand.

This chapter asks how nurses solve this ethical puzzle. Under what circumstances do they offer patients spiritual care? What kinds of therapies do they use to provide that care? I review a range of scholarly literature that points to a few possibilities. Two bodies of work—one on total institutions and another on the tensions between caregiving and professionalism—suggest some of the different ways that care professionals might think about their work. Another set of studies on identities and practices takes these insights one step further, hinting at how care professionals may translate those thoughts into actions. Synthesizing these insights, I then sketch what I call a "styles of care" framework that suggests when and how nurses care for the spiritual needs of patients. Specifically, it predicts that nurses who think of their work as a calling and value its social usefulness more than the professional and financial rewards it might bring will perceive more opportunities to dignify patients and will engage in more practices to care for them spiritually. These same workers are also predicted to apply spiritual therapies in a more methodical and systematic fashion, because doing so reinforces their self-image as socially attuned care providers. Findings support these predictions, suggesting that if caritas as a practice survives in rationalized settings, it will likely be due to a subgroup of care providers who possess a more developed "spiritual repertoire" and who view the moral demands of caritas as compatible with their true selves.

As a reminder to the reader, this book understands spiritual care as acts that honor patients' ultimate worth as human beings and that show sensitivity to their deepest, existential needs. These acts may or may not involve a reference to a transcendent being or be sanctioned by an organized religion (see also Cadge 2013; Grant, Morales, and Sallaz 2009).[2] Many aspects of patient-centered care are relatively straightforward—for example, recording patients' medical histories and dietary preferences. Spiritual care is different: it requires considerable discretion on the part of nurses because of its culturally sensitive nature. "Cultural competence," in fact, is considered central to quality patient-centered care. This type of skill may be especially tested during "unsettled" times like the present (Swidler 1986) when there is so much religious and spiritual diversity (Cadge, Ecklund, and Short 2009). By examining how nurses draw on these cultural elements in their interactions with patients, we gain new insight into the conditions under which caritas is put into action.

APPROACHING NURSES' PRACTICE OF SPIRITUAL CARE AS AN ETHICAL PUZZLE

Total Institutions and the Challenge of Dignifying Vulnerable Strangers

Since the time of Goffman's writing, scholars have observed how the moral dilemma he described in mental wards has played itself out in other care settings. Their studies provide a good point of departure for our inquiry into nurses' enactment of caritas at an academic medical center. According to these researchers, as more hospitals have adopted a business orientation, with its emphasis on centralized decision-making, cost-cutting policies, and standardized procedures, they have taken on features characteristic of total institutions (Kim et al. 2006). These features, combined with a medical model that is disease oriented and fragmented into specialties, threaten to depersonalize all patients—not just those who are diagnosed as mentally ill—and constrain hospital workers' ability to uphold their dignity (Gordon 2007).

Scholars note further that in response to complaints about the dehumanizing effects of this corporate mentality, public teaching hospitals like the one studied here have begun promoting a "detotalizing" philosophy of patient-centered care (Epstein and Street 2011). This type of care encourages nurses and other frontline personnel to improve the "quality chasm" within health organizations, not only by giving their patients a more active role in the consultation process but also by treating patients as whole persons with biological, social, psychological, and spiritual needs. Patient-centered care is consistent with a "culture change" version of human resource management that seeks to transform health organizations from "total institutions that can damage people" to safe, humane communities (Weiner and Ronch 2003) that enable patients to become self-actualized or realize their full potential.

While scholars have written extensively about the ethical quandaries these developments can pose for frontline care professionals who are expected to treat vulnerable clients as human beings while still applying impersonal therapies that treat them as objects (e.g., Stone 2000; England 2005; Glenn 2012), much less attention has been paid to how frontline personnel respond to these ethical challenges. In particular, scholars have stopped short of addressing Goffman's suggestion that the way in which care providers affirm patients' selves depends on their commitment to recreating a larger moral order or reenacting the rituals and practices of the wider society that validate the ultimate worth of individuals. A case in point is research on nurses' spiritual care. Most studies suggest that while nurses generally acknowledge that spiritual care is a part of their role and express a willingness to be involved in it, in reality, they rarely respond to patients' spiritual needs at all, or they do so on a purely ad hoc basis (McSherry 1998; Stranahan 2001). Because these inquiries rely on observational methods that are severely constrained in clinical settings, they likely have only a limited window into how and when nurses tend to patients' spiritual needs (cf. Narayanasamy and Owens 2001). They also attribute nurses' seeming lack of spiritual care to such factors as a lack of spiritual education, inadequate staffing, and the absence of links to chaplains. All these factors might play a role, but Goffman's work suggests that what matters most is how much nurses identify with their work and feel responsible for performing rituals that, outside the hospital setting, are typically used to sanctify the self.

Caregiving and Professionalism

Related research on caregiving and professionalism begins to address this issue. It focuses on the question of whether care providers can, or should, think of their work in professional terms. One strand of this literature emphasizes the vast difference between the standardized and detached care that individuals are paid to provide in the public marketplace and the spontaneous, intimate care that individuals freely receive outside it in the private sphere of family and friends (Stone 2000). According to this body of work, it is neither humanly possible nor morally desirable for care providers to try to reconcile professional and personalistic understandings of care within resource-deprived and bureaucratically driven public systems. Organizations that suggest otherwise by promoting humanistic ideologies like patient-centered care are simply trying to upgrade their image in the eyes of potential clients.

Other research questions the assumption that the public realm of money is necessarily at odds with the private domain of love (England 2005). According to this scholarship, by recognizing the myriad skills that go into providing care and reconceiving of it as a type of public good, paid care providers can begin to reconcile their professional identities with idealized notions of caregiving. Rather than viewing organizations' rhetoric about the importance of patient-centered care as mere window dressing, these studies suggest that it creates an opportunity for care workers to redefine their professional identities in more humane and morally acceptable ways.

Most recently, another body of scholarship has addressed the subject from an intersectionality perspective. This work suggests that whether paid care providers experience a conflict between professionalism and personalism or between money and love depends on the context and providers' mix of nonwork identities (Glenn 2012). It observes, for instance, that highly skilled immigrant care workers may be more motivated to embrace a professional identity within their destination country if it serves to distinguish them from lesser-skilled occupations. And depending on workers' racial, ethnic, gender, and class identities, some may view personalized care as compatible with being professional and meeting legitimate needs, whereas others may interpret it as incompatible and catering to excessive demands (Showers 2014).

This issue of whether professionalism and caregiving can coexist is especially relevant to health occupations like nursing. Although nursing was founded on a religious understanding of work that emphasized altruism and the intrinsic rewards of caring, the profession has long been secularized. At the same time, nurse academics or scholars have been some of the strongest advocates of patient-centered care, stressing the importance of addressing patients' spiritual needs. While some nurses distance themselves from angelic stereotypes by emphasizing their technical expertise (Yam 2004), others seek to preserve a sense of nursing as a calling by reclaiming Nightingale's vision of honoring the sanctity of patients as individuals (Raatikainen 1997).

Lingering Questions About the Practical Implications of Different Work Orientations

Although the preceding studies have advanced our understanding of how helping professionals conceive of their tasks and form their identities in the midst of calls for more personalized care, they rarely examine the effects of providers' work orientations on the concrete ways they practice such care and the circumstances under which they do so, which is key to understanding whether caritas as an activity that nurtures vulnerable strangers as spiritual beings is possible in scientized clinical settings. They fail to investigate the actions of care providers with different work orientations for two basic reasons.

First, these studies focus on how care providers may interpret their work differently in different situations. But it's equally likely that these providers have a stable set of dispositions toward their work. Likewise, the more scholars treat workers' identities as infinitely permeable, specialized, and changeable, the harder it is to see those identities as enforceable obligations that correlate with actual behavior (Frank and Meyer 2002).

Second, rather than studying how care providers behave, scholars focus on how they *talk* about their work experiences. Workers' conversations will sometimes contain references to specific actions they have taken to humanize their interactions with clients, such as a social worker holding the hand of child, but actions per se are rarely the subject of systematic analysis. And when they are, scholars usually focus on actions taken by workers to resist the dictates of administrators, defend their occupation's autonomy, ward off patient demands, or make what Goffman refers to as "secondary adjustments" (Goffman 1961), rather than actions that directly affirm patients' selves.

As a result of these two deficiencies, scholars gloss over the role of culture in patient-provider encounters and, in particular, the effects of more durable work orientations on decision-making and social interactions. Culture is portrayed as either a property of care providers' subjective thoughts and feelings or as an attribute of the nonwork groups to which they belong. Scholars fail, therefore, to examine the cultural challenges involved in patient-centered care that sometimes require care workers to decide which of a wide array of practices is most appropriate for dignifying the self and under which circumstances.

For example, religious institutions traditionally surrounded the self with a spiritual aura through ideas such as the soul. Rationalization has eroded this aura, and in response, a range of religious and nonreligious groups are trying to restore the spiritual qualities of self. These groups are, in a sense, competing with one another by offering different ideas of what the true nature of the human being is and how we should take care of one another spiritually. Nurses, then, become responsible for choosing which model of spiritual care to use with any given patient, and the right choice is often unclear. Religion has tried to reassert its authority over matters of the soul by, for example, stressing the importance of scripture (Emerson and Hartman 2006). Countermovements like the New Age movement advocate for more individualistic forms of spirituality (Roof 1999). (The term New Age is used here as a gloss for spiritualities not traditionally promoted by religious organizations.) And some groups have suggested that the ordinary ways in which kin express respect and concern for one another constitute forms of spiritual care (Shallenberger 1996).[3] Nurses have to engage with this ideologically charged world when faced with situations where clients' spiritual needs come to the fore. They must decide which, if any, of the practices associated with religion, the New Age movement, and family are most appropriate and when.[4] A nurse caring for a cancer patient whose condition has suddenly worsened, for example, might respond by offering prayer, giving biofeedback, holding the patient's hand, or providing no spiritual therapies at all.

Promising Developments

Fortunately, the literature on caregiving and professionalism is beginning to address these shortcomings. Scholars suggest that care providers may respond to destabilizing conditions by anchoring themselves in a particular orientation to their work. For example, Solari (2006) finds that some immigrant home care workers come to understand their caregiving in professional terms as a career, while others view it in vocational terms as a calling; which perspective they choose depends on the culture of their resettlement communities (see also Stacey 2011). What primarily motivates workers with a calling orientation is not a concern about their eternal fate (Weber 1958c) or some other religious doctrine, but the intrinsic emotional and psychological rewards they receive from enabling others to participate in or return to social life (Muirhead 2004). Also, rather than thinking that their work orientation conflicts with scientific principles, they believe that it supplements them (Raatikainen 1997). Yet other studies observe that some care providers view their work in neither professional nor vocational terms but as a form of drudgery. For instance, Sherman (2014) finds that among workers who specialize in lifestyle services (e.g., personal assistance, interior design, real estate), some deeply enjoy relating to clients, others want to help clients but maintain a professional distance from them, and still others feel overwhelmed by clients' demands and cope by focusing on mundane tasks and the pay they receive. These findings echo those of other studies (e.g., Bellah et al. 1985) that show that most people think of their work in one of three ways: as a meaningful calling, as a career that brings them status, or as a job that helps them meet their financial needs.

Several researchers have also begun exploring the possibility that, depending on their work orientations, some helping professionals may be more motivated than others to embrace their company's humanistic ideals. Lopez (2006) finds, for example, that certain health care facilities provide workers with the resources needed to personalize care and help patients to construct or maintain a viable self. And even when facilities do not, though, some workers will still speak of their commitment to treating patients with dignity. Unlike those who view the profane conditions of today's care environments as threats to the self, these workers frame such conditions as presenting opportunities to affirm both their own selves and those of their patients.

This body of work helps us to better understand how care providers may develop stable work orientations. But to understand how their orientation to work connects with their actual caregiving, we need to bring in two additional sets of literature: identity theory and practice theory. The first helps us to see that the way in which individuals view themselves influences how they understand their social roles. The second ties this understanding with action. Putting these different strands of research in dialogue provides a groundwork for understanding whether, when, and how caregivers put spirituality into action.

Identity and Practice Perspectives

Identity theorists (Burke and Stets 2009; Stets and Carter 2012) share with Goffman several assumptions about the self and its identities. Ultimately, in their view, the self is developed through social interaction: as we observe other people, respond to their opinions about ourselves, and internalize those opinions, we get a sense of who we are. To successfully participate in society, we need other people to affirm our sense of self, and we also need to affirm our own sense of who we are. Our sense of ourselves also has multiple parts. We have more than one identity, and each identity is tied to one of our social roles; for example, someone may identify as a sister, a leader, and a nurse, each of which speaks to a role she plays in others' lives. But these roles aren't our identities; our identities are the *meanings* we attach to our roles. So our answers to questions like "What does it mean to be a nurse?" are what gives us our sense of self (Schwalbe 1993). Some people's social positions allow them to assign meanings to others' roles and tell people how to enact their roles. For example, hospital administrators are in a position to tell nurses to be both professional and personal when they care for patients. But even then, those meanings and prescriptions are up for negotiation, because just as society shapes our sense of self, we shape society (Stryker 1980).

Identity theory, however, departs from Goffman in significant ways. Goffman suggests that identities are fluid and undifferentiated, producing a situational self that individuals strategically display to others like actors playing out a script. Identity scholars, on the other hand, presume that identities are relatively permanent and ranked in prominence to reflect an "ideal self" that individuals seek out situations to verify. Goffman characterizes society as basically tentative in nature and always in the process of being created and interpreted. In contrast, identity theorists suggest that society is structured and defined by patterned behavior.

Sociological research on practices (Bourdieu 1977) complements this approach to identity in addressing the linkages between individuals' behavior and society at large. It argues that when individuals enter organizational settings like hospitals, they carry with them repertoires of actions learned in their everyday lives—what Bourdieu calls their habitus—that they seek out opportunities to deploy. So, for example, when nurses face a situation at work that may pose a threat to a patient's sense of self—for example, a frightening medical prognosis—they'll respond by drawing on their culturally prescribed dispositions or toolkits. One nurse's toolkit may include active listening and prayer, while another's may include soothing touch and meditation, depending on what they've drawn from their culture. These practices then serve as cultural bridges to outside environments for both the nurse and the patient.

STYLES OF CARE

To conceptualize how caregivers put caritas into action, I draw on these bodies of work to outline a model of *styles of care*. In this model, the rationalization of modern care organizations threatens to defame the selves of care recipients (figure 6.1). But when organizations adopt humanizing ideologies such as "holistic care" or "spirituality in health care," this threat can be reduced. Humanizing ideologies can be either ceremonial in nature, in which case organizations only pay lip service to an idea, or tangible, in

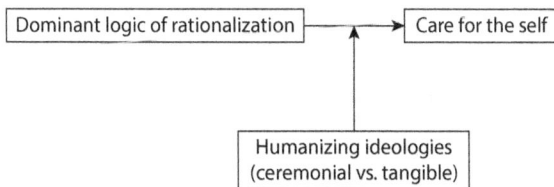

FIGURE 6.1. Styles of care: rationalization, humanizing ideologies, and care for the self.

which case they put it into practice. During periods of heightened accountability like the present, however, hospitals and other care organizations are under pressure to "put their money where their mouth is," so to speak, and to really act on the humanizing ideologies they espouse.

Administrators and other organizational leaders can help render humanizing ideologies more tangible by providing various resources, but succeeding in this endeavor ultimately depends on the practices of frontline care workers (figure 6.2). Because these workers interact with clients directly, translating ideologies into acts of care is typically their responsibility. This responsibility is especially challenging when the larger society is fragmented into the worldviews of competing groups that have different ideas about the specific circumstances under which the self, including the spiritual self, needs to be honored and with what substantive practices. For example, religious groups may suggest that when caring for a sick individual who is a member of a church, the laying on of hands is an appropriate practice. In contrast, New Age groups may advise that when any ill person is struggling to sleep, therapeutic touch should be applied.

Workers will respond differently to this fragmentation depending on their work orientations. Some workers will be highly motivated to seek out circumstances to care for others and will deploy a wide range of care practices, both because they find them intrinsically rewarding and because they align with their ideal sense of self (see Burke and Stets 2009; Stets and Carter 2012).[5] In particular, workers who identify most closely with their role as a calling will perceive more opportunities and engage in more acts

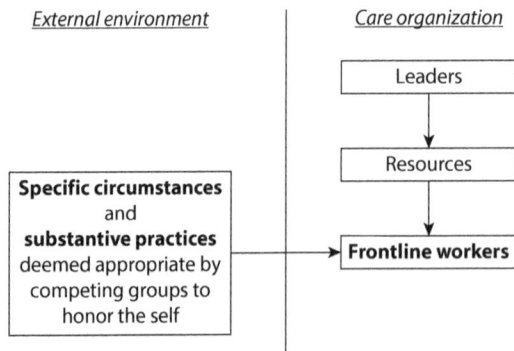

FIGURE 6.2. Styles of care: rendering humanizing ideologies tangible.

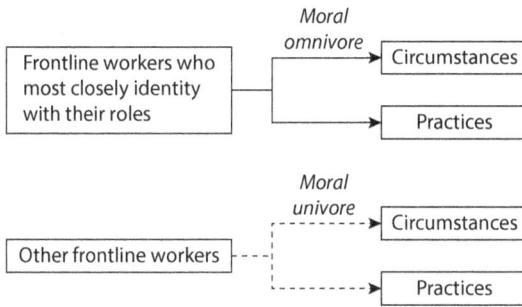

FIGURE 6.3. Styles of care: moral omnivore versus moral univore.

to affirm clients' dignity (Stets and Carter 2012). These care workers, then, will act more like moral omnivores, who possess a diverse repertoire of moral solutions, than moral univores, who possess a less varied repertoire, because in affirming the selves of multiple others, workers with callings affirm their own identities as well (figure 6.3).

Workers' styles of care are defined not just by the number of circumstances they respond to and the number of practices they deploy, but also the degree to which they selectively apply practices to circumstances (figure 6.4). Workers who distance themselves from their roles by defining them as careers or jobs tend to apply practices in a more random fashion, a pattern typical of moral bricoleurs, who use whatever resources are available. In contrast, those who most strongly self-identify with their roles as a calling do so more methodically; they resemble moral engineers who select

Frontline workers who most closely identify with their roles

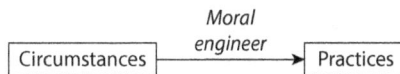

Other frontline workers

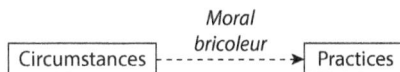

FIGURE 6.4. Styles of care: moral engineer versus moral bricoleur.

what are considered the best resources because, again, their action reinforces their self-conceptions as deeply sensitive care providers.[6]

Why, When, and How Nurses Practice Spiritual Care Differently

These arguments suggest that nurses' work orientations will influence when and how they care for patients' selves. Stated more formally, I would predict that:

1) Nurses who think of their work as a calling will see more opportunities to provide spiritual care than nurses who consider their work a career or job.
2) Nurses who think of their work as a calling are more likely to engage in spiritual care practices than those who consider their work a career or job.

And, depending on how much they identify with their work as a calling, some nurses will be more thoughtful and systematic about how they choose which spiritual care practices to use in in which situations. Specifically, we would expect that:

3) Nurses who think of their work as a calling will deploy spiritual interventions in a less random fashion than nurses who consider their work a career or job.

METHODS

To assess these predictions, I compiled a list of circumstances that might require spiritual interventions and a list of therapies that might be considered spiritual in nature. The lists were created during a focus group session and were based on the opinions of ten nurses and five professors from University Hospital's nursing school. Bedside nurses were then asked in the survey to state in which of the 40 circumstances they would likely suggest, offer, or provide spiritual care to a patient. And they were asked which of the 24 spiritual therapies they had ever suggested, offered, or provided to a patient (see appendix to chapter 6 for a description of these items and the analytical strategy).

I decided that a survey was better suited to assessing nurses' styles of care than interviews or observations because it would allow me to systematically analyze how nurses with different work orientations apply different types of practices to different types of situations. The fact that the survey explicitly asked nurses whether they had ever suggested, offered, or provided certain practices also suggested that the survey items captured actual as opposed to hypothetical practices. Note, however, that the survey items did not ask respondents whether they themselves thought specific practices were spiritual or not. Rather, the goal was to determine which of the practices identified by nursing scholars as spiritual or potentially spiritual were deployed by respondents. Readers need to keep this point in mind when interpreting the results that follow, since it means, for example, that while some nurses may provide aroma therapy to patients or hold their hand, not all of them would necessarily consider these practices "spiritual."

Three measures of work orientation were employed, labeled *calling*, *career*, and *job*. In the survey, nurses were asked to indicate which of the following statements best describes their present attitude about their work as a nurse: "My work is a calling" (I do what I do because I think it is personally fulfilling and socially useful); "My work is a career" (I do what I do because it provides opportunities for professional advancement); and "My work is a job" (I do what I do because of the financial rewards). Answers to these questions were coded as 1 = Yes and 0 = No.

THE VARIED WAYS THAT NURSES PRACTICE SPIRITUAL CARE

Table 6.1 shows that virtually all bedside nurses think that spiritual resources should be made available to patients when they explicitly request them or face serious and emotionally difficult situations. Roughly half of nurses think that spiritual interventions are warranted when patients are in denial, have lost their composure, and are experiencing physical pain. A smaller percentage of nurses think that the remaining circumstances (e.g., a patient struggles to sleep, a patient won't eat) call for spiritual intervention.

Table 6.2 reveals that of the 24 spiritual therapies, 5 had been recommended or employed by a majority of bedside nurses: holding a patient's hand, listening, laughing, praying, and being present with a patient. A third to little less than half of nurses have offered massages, therapeutic touch, music therapy, guided imagery, and meditation. The remaining therapies have been used by a minority of nurses (under 30 percent).

TABLE 6.1

Percentage of nurses who would offer, suggest, or provide spiritual help when a patient...

Circumstance	Percent
Explicitly requests spiritual support	98
Is about to die	96
Is grieving	93
Receives bad news	93
Is crying	86
Asks about the meaning of life	82
Often prays or seems close to God	81
Seems depressed	78
Is a victim of abuse	75
Is expecting to be healed by God	74
Is a member of a church, or other religious organization	71
Is about to go to surgery	70
Is suicidal	69
Is at the hospital during a holiday season	67
Is alienated from friends and family	67
Is angry at God	65
Is having marital conflict or family conflict	64
Feels guilty	62
Has few visitors	62
Is experiencing a loss of identity	59
Has been upset by his or her visitors	58
Is in denial	54
Has lost his or her composure	50
Is unconscious	48
Is experiencing physical pain	46
Receives good news	45
Suffers from addictions	44
Seems unwilling to forgive	41
Is angry at organized religion	41
Struggles to sleep	35
Questions the effectiveness of medicine	34
Is not a member of a church or other religious organization	32
Doesn't interact with staff	32
Is appreciative of staff	31
Is angry at staff	30
Won't cooperate with treatment	29
Complains more than usual	26
Is disoriented	24
Won't eat	23
Is placing too many demands on staff	22

TABLE 6.2
Spiritual therapies that nurses have offered, suggested, or provided to patients

Therapy	Percent
Holding a patient's hand	92
Listening	92
Laughing	84
Praying	71
Being present with a patient	62
Massage	49
Therapeutic touch	43
Music therapy	38
Guided imagery	36
Meditation	34
Spiritual counseling	29
Scripture reading	26
Religious sacraments	24
Laying on of hands	21
Sacred music	20
Worship	18
Aromatherapy	14
Centering	14
Energy work	9
Biofeedback	8
Acupuncture	7
Chanting	4
Fasting	4
Repatterning	2

As mentioned earlier and reported again in table 6.3, most nurses surveyed view their work in purely secular terms as a career (60 percent) or a job (17 percent). Nonetheless, consistent with prior studies (Raatikainen 1997), a fairly substantial percentage (23 percent) consider their work a calling. Unlike individuals who labeled their work a calling during the time of Calvin, however, nurses who embrace this work orientation are no more likely to attend religious services or identify themselves as religious than others performing the same work.

TABLE 6.3
Descriptive statistics on work orientations

	Calling (23%)	Career (60%)	Job (17%)
Attend religious services at least monthly (1 = Yes)	37%	36%	35%
I consider myself a religious person (1 = Yes)	44%	37%	50%
Work satisfaction (4 = Very Satisfied . . . 1 = Very Unsatisfied)	3.41*	3.28	2.88*
I am skilled at gaining the trust of patients (1 = Yes)	87%*	76%	76%
Feelings of inauthenticity[a]	2.06*	2.24	2.33

Note: Total number of nurses in sample = 299. * Indicates whether a group's mean score is significantly different from those of the other two groups.

[a] Scale composed of two items that ask respondents how strongly they agree or disagree with the statements "I often feel I cannot be myself at work" or "I often have to fake how I really feel at work." Respondents who score low on this scale experience fewer feelings of inauthenticity.

Instead, what distinguishes nurses with callings are their more positive self-feelings. Specifically, they are significantly more likely than those with careers or jobs to express overall satisfaction with their work, which is characteristic of more intrinsically motivated employees. Calling nurses are also significantly more likely to have confidence in their ability to gain patients' trust and significantly less likely to suffer from feelings of inauthenticity. These findings comport with the contemporary understanding of calling as work that is both personally rewarding and socially useful. They also suggest that what motivates nurses with callings is the greater emotional intensity they experience when caring for the selves of others (Collins 2004).

In the analyses that follow, we explore the implications of these work orientations for when and how nurses perform spiritual care.

Circumstances Said to Warrant Spiritual Interventions

Table 6.4 tests the prediction that nurses with callings are more apt to identify situations as warranting spiritual interventions. Instead of examining what the three types of nurses think about each of the 40 circumstances listed in table 6.1, table 6.4 breaks down these circumstances into four basic types—situations involving patients who are uncooperative (e.g., they complain more than usual), patients who are in dire straits (e.g., they are suicidal), patients who appear religious (e.g., they bring a Bible with

TABLE 6.4
Responses of nurses to circumstances that warrant spiritual help

	Uncooperative patient	Patient in dire straits	Religious patient	Angry patient
Nurses with callings	+	+	+	
Nurses with careers			+	

them), and patients who are angry (e.g., they are mad at God). Table 6.4 also reports whether nurses with callings or career orientations are more likely to deem these four circumstances as needing spiritual interventions than nurses who have the least personal attachment to their work and consider it simply a job. In this table and the two that follow, a plus sign indicates that nurses with a calling or career work orientation are significantly more apt to think that a type of circumstance warrants spiritual help than those with a job orientation, and a minus sign indicates the opposite. Blanks indicate that there is no significant difference between nurses in terms of whether they view a circumstance as requiring spiritual help. (Results control for other characteristics of nurses, such as age and gender, and each nurse's typical patients, such as how long their patients typically stay in the hospital.)

Findings reveal that nurses with callings are significantly more likely to interpret situations involving uncooperative patients as needing spiritual care. Nurses with callings are also more likely to perceive that such care is needed with patients who are in dire straits. And calling nurses (as well as career nurses) more often think that spiritual care is appropriate with patients who seem religious than do job nurses. Situations involving patients who are angry are the only ones that calling nurses are not more likely to perceive as warranting spiritual care. In general, then, results support the prediction that nurses with callings view more situations as requiring spiritual interventions.[7]

Spiritual Therapies Deployed

Table 6.5 tests the prediction that nurses with callings apply a wider range of spiritual therapies. Here we break down the 24 therapies shown in Table 6.2 into three basic types—those associated with the New Age

TABLE 6.5
Types of spiritual therapies that nurses with callings and careers have suggested, offered, or provided to patients

	New Age	Religious	Familial
Nurses with callings	+	+	+
Nurses with careers			

movement (e.g., biofeedback), organized religion (e.g., prayer), and practices commonly performed by family members or close friends (e.g., holding another's hand). Findings reveal that nurses who identify with their work as a calling are significantly more likely to apply all three types of therapies—New Age, religious, and familial—than their job counterparts (as indicated by the plus signs in the second row). In contrast, there are no significant differences between career and job nurses in their use of spiritual therapies (as indicated by the blanks in the third row).[8] All told, table 6.5 provides uniform support for the prediction that calling nurses are more likely to engage in spiritual care practices.

Matching Spiritual Therapies to Circumstances

Having determined that nurses with callings perceive more circumstances requiring spiritual intervention and have a broader repertoire of spiritual therapies, I next assess the prediction that workers with callings will deploy therapies in response to situational prompts in a less random fashion. Table 6.6 provides a detailed analysis of the types of practices that nurses with different work orientations are significantly more likely to use under various types of circumstances. A plus sign indicates that nurses with a particular work orientation are significantly more likely to use a certain type of practice under a certain type of circumstance, a minus sign indicates the opposite, and a blank indicates that no relationship exists between those types of practices and circumstances. Panel A of table 6.6 reveals that nurses who consider their work a calling are significantly more likely to refrain from selecting New Age therapies when caring for patients facing dire circumstances and significantly more likely to choose such therapies when patients are angry. Calling nurses are more likely to apply religious therapies when dealing with seemingly religious patients. And they resist

TABLE 6.6
Nurses' selection of spiritual therapies

	New Age	Religious	Familial
Panel A: Nurses with callings			
Uncooperative patients			−
Patients in dire straits	−		+
Patients wanting religious services		+	
Angry patients	+		
Panel B: Nurses with careers			
Uncooperative patients			
Patients in dire straits	+		
Patients wanting religious services		+	
Angry patients			
Panel C: Nurses with jobs			
Uncooperative patients			
Patients in dire straits			
Patients wanting religious services		+	
Angry patients			−

using familial therapies when dealing with uncooperative patients but resort to them when treating patients whose circumstances are dire.

In contrast, panels B and C suggest that other nurses select spiritual therapies more haphazardly. The therapies of nurses with careers and jobs are statistically associated with fewer types of circumstances and, in some cases, none at all. Career nurses are likely to employ New Age therapies when comforting patients in dire straits and religious therapies when treating more religious patients, but their use of familial therapies is unrelated to any patient circumstance. Similarly, job nurses are prone to apply religious therapies to religious patients and less likely to apply familial therapies to angry patients, but they do not apply New Age therapies to any particular set of circumstances.

Table 6.7 summarizes how the effects of circumstances on nurses' selection of spiritual therapies vary depending on whether nurses relate to work as a calling, a career, or a job. Uppercase letters indicate that, for a particular work orientation, a certain set of circumstances had a significant

TABLE 6.7
Work orientations of nurses who select spiritual therapies

	New Age	Religious	Familial
Uncooperative patients			**Calling**
Patients in dire straits	**Calling** **CAREER**		CALLING
Patients wanting religious services		CALLING CAREER JOB	
Angry patients	**CALLING**		Job

Note: Uppercase letters indicate that, for a particular work orientation, a certain set of circumstances had a significant positive effect on a certain set of practices. Lowercase letters indicate that, for a particular work orientation, a certain set of circumstances had a significant negative effect on a certain set of practices. If a work orientation is also in bold type, this indicates that its associated effect or slope coefficient is significantly different than for either of the other two groups.

positive effect on a certain set of practices. Lowercase letters indicate that, for a particular work orientation, a certain set of circumstances had a significant negative effect on a certain set of practices. If a work orientation is also in bold type, its associated effect is significantly different than for either of the other two groups.

Table 6.7 reveals that only three of the nine statistically significant relationships reported in table 6.6 are common to all nurses: nurses with callings, careers, and jobs each use religious therapies when patients want religious services. The majority (four) of the remaining six relationships are unique to calling nurses. Specifically, nurses who see their work as a calling are significantly more likely than those who see it as a career or job to avoid New Age practices in dire situations but to employ them in ones involving anger. They are also significantly less likely to use familial practices when patients' cooperation is at stake but to use them when circumstances are dire. In short, findings suggest that nurses who see their work as a calling have more distinctive styles of care and are more methodical and discriminate. These nurses seem to behave like moral engineers: they target the remedy to the problem.

CONCLUSION

"The spiritual" is an open concept: it's broad enough that people can define it in different ways. It's also in tension with rationalist principles that cast doubt on its reality. These two realities mean that when today's care facilities promote a "biopsychosocial-spiritual" model of care, frontline staff need to negotiate between these competing ideas as they figure out how to put that model into practice. This negotiation, as well as the additional responsibility, likely puts extra work on their plate and requires extra commitment from them (Saad, de Medeiros, and Mosini 2017).

Existing perspectives on public religion provide little insight into who is most likely to make spiritual care happen, when will they do so, and how. Secularization scholars contend that rationalization suppresses the vocational ethic and any sense of work as a calling. They argue that bureaucracies and science disconnect secular spheres from the religious sphere, which reduces religion to a matter of individual conscience and creates inconsistencies between people's private beliefs and their public actions (Chaves 2010). Lived religion scholars disagree; they argue that spiritual practices can help people can bring spiritual meaning into their larger lives. These practices might be traditional religious practices like prayer and scripture reading, or they might be practices more closely associated with the New Age movement like guided imagery and energy work. Regardless of which spiritual tradition they're associated with, the key point is that the spiritual practice evokes a transcendent or "more than ordinary" experience that reminds people of commitments and possibilities beyond those of the rationalized world (Ammerman 2014). But these scholars' focus is firmly on how spiritual practice can cultivate and sacralize one's "inner self." They stop short of explaining what role, if any, spiritual practices might play in sanctifying the selves of strangers.

This chapter sought to advance our understanding of the pragmatics of caritas by outlining a framework for studying hospital workers' different styles of caring for patients' spiritual needs. Consistent with its expectations, findings reveal that nurses who consider their work a calling interpret a broader range of situations as warranting spiritual intervention and deploy a larger set of spiritual practices to care for patients' selves. They also apply practices to situations more selectively. This finding suggests that these workers' personal investment in their role facilitates creative navigation of the constraints and opportunities at work. In contrast, nurses who consider their work a job or career perceive fewer opportunities and use fewer practices. And they apply practices to situations in a largely random fashion. This finding would imply that nurses who view their labor as a job are less knowledgeable about how and when spiritual norms are to be practiced. Those with careers seem more familiar with such norms but not so committed to them that they apply them systematically (Pache and Santos 2013). In short, how, when, and with what degree of nuance caritas is enacted in a scientific environment hinges on whether this religious ethic's moral demands resonate with nurses' work identities.

Findings underscore how spirituality is not a fixed or achieved state but a meaning that is variously acted upon depending on the social situation (Kucinskas et al. 2017). Similarly, they suggest that identities are more than devices that organize the self. They can be stratagems that helping professionals apply to affirm both their own and others' sense of self. At the same time, it is important not to attribute nurses' varied spiritual care simply to their self-identities. As shown in the previous chapter (see table 5.1), whether nurses can believe their work is a calling depends on factors like the severity of their patients' conditions, whether the technology they use frightens patients, and whether they have supportive coworkers. In these and other ways, nurses' ability to think and act as if their care is a calling is rooted in a broader social context.

Finally, this chapter's analyses speak to the fact that although they may be in the minority, care workers with callings may nonetheless function as "internal activists" (Meyerson 2003). These tempered radicals strongly identify with the scientific role their hospital has assigned to them but are also deeply committed to preserving caritas as a practical possibility by creatively enacting sacred rituals drawn from the wider society. This meaning-making role is often overlooked by scholars who portray front-line employees as largely passive actors who simply pay lip service to their organization's ideals (Meyer and Rowan 1977).

While this analysis makes important contributions, it is also open to criticism. Some might fault it for not examining whether the practices studied here are, in fact, beneficial to patients. That is, in caring for patients' spiritual needs, nurses could, as Goffman (1961) also suggested, infringe on the selves of patients. Others might argue that its findings have little relevance beyond nursing, which is unique in the extent to which it directly cares for others. And some might object that in comparison to the administrative and technical tasks performed within hospitals, the kinds of practices examined here are too informal and minimalist to be socially relevant.

With respect to the first criticism, it is true that nurses who construe their work as a calling might abuse their power over patients and seek to proselytize or otherwise abuse them. However, our findings indicate that calling nurses' interpretations of religious situations and use of religious practices cannot be explained by their allegiance to religious organizations. They are no more likely to attend religious services than nurses with careers and jobs. Also, if spiritual care is being used as a cover to exploit patients or is being applied in culturally incompetent ways (Sullivan et al. 2015), as a few nurses in this study raised concerns about (and will be discussed in the next chapter), it is all the more important to do what was done here and study nurses' styles of care. By specifying which combinations of tactics and circumstances lend themselves to the exploitation of patients, we can better understand not only how ideologies are used to manipulate the ill, but also the subtle, biased treatment of disadvantaged groups (Lockhart and Danis 2010).

Hospital nurses are not the only health care workers who provide direct care; home care providers, hospice teams, and other health care workers might use some of the same care techniques that the nurses I studied use (e.g., Stacey 2011). Teachers, social workers, and other helping professionals don't work with people whose lives are literally at stake, but they do often work with vulnerable strangers, and they certainly face some of the same cultural challenges that hospital nurses face. Like nurses, these workers are under growing pressure both to standardize their tasks and to customize them to provide a more student- or client-centered experience. They may not be expected to provide spiritual care, but they may be required to expand their skill sets, increase their cultural competence, and care for other people's selves in new ways, all of which may be difficult for those who understand their work primarily in terms of status or money.

Although the practices investigated here are ones that may not fit bureaucratic definitions of "real work," the same is true of many forms of care, such as parenting, on which societal functioning depends (England 2005). Also, as Goffman (1961) would suggest, personalistic care upholds the idea that we all do have a unique self and that that matters. Personalized care carves out a moral space that enables people to be validated as intrinsically precious beings. While this kind of care may not result in large-scale institutional change, it may change organizational cultures in less conspicuous ways: it may function as a "provisional institution" or a temporary solution that mitigates the suffering brought on by technical and bureaucratic systems (Lawrence, Suddaby, and Leca 2011).

Finally, in addition to providing new insights into when and how caritas can stick in scientized settings of care, findings speak to some practical problems surrounding patient-centered care. Proponents of the this care suggest that frontline workers like nurses want to be unburdened from the drudgery of productivity-driven, assembly-line medicine so that they can address patients' deeper needs, including those of an emotional, social, or spiritual nature (Epstein and Street 2011). Yet, as results here indicate, some nurses may be more motivated to do so than others. Although such differences were not an issue in the past, today they could be as hospitals are being publicly graded on their patient-centered care on websites like the Centers for Medicare and Medicaid Services (www.cms.gov) and scrutinized on others like Zocdoc (www.zocdoc.com) and Yelp (www.yelp.com). In addition to demanding that all nurses be more productive and efficient, therefore, administrators may expect them to be committed and culturally competent providers of patient-centered care. Nurses who self-identify with their work as a calling may welcome such an expectation and feel equipped to meet it, while others may view it as less compatible with their true selves and beyond their skill set.

Of course, under some circumstances, the specific spiritual interventions implemented by caregivers may be less important to patients than whether they receive any spiritual comfort at all—whether others are helping them retain a sense of being intrinsically valuable in circumstances that seem almost designed to rob them of their human dignity. This is how I felt, at least, shortly after my transplant procedure.

Doug was right.

Although I tried to dismiss his earlier comments about postsurgery pain, it turns out to be torturous. The pain is tolerable for the first few minutes after I awake and am told by the tending nurse that the surgery has gone well. Immediately afterwards, I also meet—for the first time— the chief surgeon, Amadeo Marcos. He inspects my incisions without saying a word. Satisfied with his handiwork and apparently wanting me to look as neat as his sutures, he orders the nurse to shave my facial hair.

But the pain grows soon after he exits the room, and judging from the concerned look of family members gathered around me, something

is not quite right. I am bent over in pain; when sitting up in my bed, I see what I believe is a bright light shining behind me. I ask the nurses to close the curtains to stop the sun's glare but am told there is nothing behind me but a solid wall. As the cramping and delirium intensify, my family are increasingly worried and reluctant to touch me. They stand back, looking as helpless as I felt years ago in my role as a chaplain when visiting the mother of a drowned child and realizing I had nothing in my toolkit that was suitable for the moment. My youngest daughter, who is four, becomes so upset that she kicks a physician assistant for what she and the surgical team have apparently done to me. The rest of my family maintain a worried and careful distance from my bed, while she screams until she is allowed to approach me and rest her small hand on my forearm.

I begin thinking I have been the victim of a terrible lie, that the doctors knew my odds of a healthy recovery were low but were sympathetic to our family's circumstances and took a chance anyway. A nurse assures me that my father has survived the procedure and is recovering in a room three floors below me, but I cannot help but think the seriousness of his condition is being understated as well. I overhear my aunt whisper to my mom that she caught a brief glimpse of my dad shortly after he was wheeled out of surgery and that his face is swollen to the point of being unrecognizable. Doug's theatrical account of patients' postsurgical experiences now seems, if anything, to downplay the gravity of the situation.

Fortunately, by the fourth day, the pain starts to subside. Dr. Marcos also orders me to begin standing and taking small steps so that I might soon visit my dad downstairs and see for myself that he is improving. By the sixth day, when I can shuffle up and down the hallway on my own, I am no longer overcome by feelings of panic but of determination to verify that my dad is okay.

My entire family accompany me on the journey from my room to my dad's. My wife, mom, sister, aunt, and three daughters feel more comfortable touching me now as we squeeze into an elevator together. Pent-up feelings begin to surface. Some cry and laugh, while others become edgy and bicker, but our bond is palpable.

On the way down, we stop on the main floor, where I go into the hospital's gift shop and purchase for each of our three daughters a plush animal—an elephant for Natasha, a turtle for Allison, and a frog for Kelsey. From there we go back to the elevator and descend to the basement, where my dad is staying. We pass the room of an Egyptian dignitary who, according to the nurse leading us, was flown in the night before for a cadaveric liver transplant, a reminder of our own desperation and privilege.

When we arrive at my dad's room, he is seated asleep on his bed. His face and most of his upper torso are inflamed and bloated. I now understand why others were hesitant to approach me earlier—I, too, looked like a mess after the procedure. But as he awakens, looking startled and seeing us all for the first time in a week, we draw close to him and softly reassure him that he got through the procedure okay. Our family members then use the same "spiritual therapy" my youngest daughter applied to me—we each reach out and gently touch his arm.

Chapter Seven

BRIDGING SCIENCE AND SPIRITUALITY THROUGH STORYTELLING

*As I became more attuned to the subtle ways that nurses upheld patients'
dignity, I grew interested in how they might describe those encounters. Our
stories reveal our understandings, and I wondered what their stories would
reveal about how they understood the relationship between spirituality and
modern medicine. Because their hospital promoted spirituality as a vague,
open-ended concept, they would have to compose those narratives from
scratch, which also made me curious about how they, as storytellers, rendered
their experiences with patients and convinced themselves that the spiritual
was or was not compatible with medical science. Weber feared that spiritually informed care would conflict with care workers' scientific training. Would
nurses agree with him? Or would they figure out ways to portray the two
kinds of care as agreeable?*

*Meanwhile, my six-month residency as a chaplain intern was drawing to
a close. I had begun the internship convinced that the chaplaincy was important, and I was even thinking about making a career change. But it wasn't
long before I began to have doubts. The program's promotional materials
described chaplains as playing a critical role in patients' well-being. But in
reality, we seemed to occupy a marginal and awkward place in the hospital.
The staff chaplain seemed to share my experience. "In most instances," he told
me, "you never know for sure if your services are really wanted." And because
the hospital faced unrelenting pressure to shorten patient stays, chaplains had*

only fleeting opportunities to develop relationships with patients and address their spiritual needs. Typically, a chaplain was paged for help when a patient was preparing for surgery, when the trauma team needed someone to contact a family member, when staff members were too busy with technical matters to chat with a lonely patient, or when staff members found comfort in having a religious figure in their midst during an emergency. Some of these occasions could be quite meaningful, but they were few and far between, at least during the hours I worked. On average, I was paged just four times during each of my twelve-hour night shifts. I spent the rest of my time sleeping, checking out the cafeteria's vending machines for a snack, or wandering the hallways and chatting with janitors mopping the floors.

I also discovered that the well-being of patients, their families, and staff rarely hinged on my response. At first, I thought it might. I struggled during my night shifts to sleep in the chaplain's on-call quarters, fearing that I would not awaken or would be late intervening in a crisis. But after learning that there were few situations in which chaplains were urgently needed, I became less anxious and calibrated my actions. Instead of panicking when I received a late-night call from the ER, for instance, I would often pause and remind myself that my most important contribution would be to exhibit calmness. Instead of rushing to be with a patient who received a terminal cancer diagnosis, I would first read sections of the Dictionary of Pastoral Care and Counseling *to better understand the mourning process and determine what help I might offer. And rather than trying to muster up saintly answers to spiritual questions, I would focus on listening to patients and not pretending I had the authority to make sense of their tragedies.*

More than anything, I learned that the staff members that patients most often turned to for spiritual comfort were not chaplains, as the director of the Clinical Pastoral Education (CPE) program claimed, but those closest at hand—bedside nurses. In fact, throughout the CPE program I, too, turned to nurses for advice. Some of the wiser ones seemed to know when a visit from a chaplain would be helpful and how the chaplain could help.

On one occasion I was summoned to the newborn intensive care unit (NICU) to meet with parents who had received "bad news." Before buzzing for entry into the unit and while washing my hands with antibacterial soap, I studied the crayon drawings of grateful survivors hung above the doorway. There were mashups of smiling, stick-figured doctors and nurses and rainbowed worlds of home, family, and pets that these children could be with as a result of the staff's efforts. When the electronic latch and door opened, three nurses dressed in similarly designed blouses with childlike images of toys, cats, and dogs hurriedly made their way out, crying. The sole nurse who remained inside gestured for me to follow her. All of the pods had their curtains drawn open, their incubators still and empty, with the exception of the one in the most distant corner of the room. We passed a team of surgeons. Not acknowledging our presence, they wrapped their metallic instruments in sterile cloths of white with the solemnity of a ritual.

I heard what sounded like a soft chant coming from behind the curtain of the last pod. The nurse slowly moved aside its curtain. Inside, a woman with her back to us was huddled over. Opposite her was a man in tears, murmuring some song about little angels returning to heaven. When the nurse touched the woman on her shoulder, the woman turned, revealing an abnormally small and thin baby in her lap. Its skin was a ghastly purple with visible veins. Streams of blood ran from both of its nostrils. I recoiled and planted myself, feeling I could only observe from a distance. But the nurse nudged me forward. Gently grasping my right arm, she guided and placed it on the mother's shoulder. I silently held it there until the nurse, with a look of approval, signaled that it was time for me to exit. That same nurse told me later that day that the moment she stopped being disturbed by others' suffering was the day she would quit her profession.

Incidents like that one in the NICU continued to disturb me, but my confidence in dealing with them slowly grew to the point where I felt I had achieved at least a craft-level mastery of chaplaincy. And by doing as one nurse suggested and recording some of my experiences with patients as stories, I began to make sense of events that at the time often made little sense, and I began to understand how spirituality fit into health care. But sometime around the sixth month of the chaplaincy program I felt it was time for a change. I began reverting to some of my secular habits as a sociologist, distancing myself to better understand the social context I had observed and experienced. In particular, during the downtimes of my nightly shifts, I started composing questions about the place of spirituality in nurses' work that I had wondered about during my time as a chaplain, questions that would eventually be included in a survey that I administered at the hospital after my time as a chaplain intern.

My last patient encounter—number 99—was perhaps a fitting ending to my time as chaplain, although the one preceding it was more memorable and haunting. As my shift was ending and I was about to exit the ER, an intoxicated patient who had been shot in the rear and was lying on a stretcher noticed me passing by. He immediately threw off his bedsheet and mooned me, saying, "Here's to you, buddy." Not wanting to be embroiled in an argument just before stepping down, I saluted him and continued on my way.

My mind was also elsewhere. I had just spent the previous two hours in the ER trying to contact the local relatives of an undocumented worker. His left leg had been severed while he'd been trying to hop a train from Nogales to Tucson. The surgical team had tried to reattach the leg, but thirty minutes into the procedure they'd discovered that it was two inches shorter than the right one. Another section of the left leg had apparently been excised but was not included in the bloody bag that was flown in with the worker. The ambulance crew didn't have any information about the missing part either. At the time my shift ended, the team had still not decided what, if anything, could be done about the leg. The room was speechless. As I departed, the chief surgeon glanced upward at the ceiling and then bowed his head with a heavy sigh.

Later he and the other staff would probably spend time processing the experience. I wondered how they would understand what they witnessed, how they would put this tragedy into words. Would they view the event through the bloodless logic of modern medicine as just another body that regretfully could not be repaired? Or would they think there was something more valuable at stake and was perhaps lost in this stranger? What would they conclude about the relationship between science and the spiritual? And how might they fashion a story about this event that, in their minds at least, made that conclusion compelling?

When we're exposed to suffering, we can long to escape mundane reality and find otherworldly understandings of life. I saw this in the NICU and wherever patients and their loved ones were confronting the reality of death. But it can be hard for people to share these deeply moral experiences in modern settings like hospitals, where the language of science rules. That's how I understood the surgical team's horrified silence before the helpless undocumented worker.

Weber spoke about science muffling spiritual yearnings in one of his last public lectures, titled "Science as Vocation" and given in 1919. He told his audience that we live in a time of "disenchantment" when "there are no mysterious incalculable forces that come into play" (Weber 1958e, 139). Modern society, he argued, is guided instead by the core belief "that one can, in principle, master all things by calculation" (139). Weber was no Luddite about the benefits of advanced technology, but he was also keenly aware of what had been lost in the disenchantment of the world. He worried that modern people had lost access to "meanings that go beyond the merely practical and technical" (139). He, like Tolstoy, doubted that science could ever answer the only question that really matters: "What shall we do and how shall we live?" (143).

Weber did not live long enough to fully explore the ways the world might be reenchanted. The closest he came was to suggest that it might require a mass charismatic renewal. But he also hinted at another possibility—that mundane, everyday existence might be reenchanted, or recover the sense of awe and mystery traditionally provided by religion, through narrative. As Arthur Frank (2002) later explained, Weber thought that telling stories about their lives is one way people confront the reality of disenchantment, make their experiences understandable to themselves and others, and align their actions with the things that matter most to them. Simply put, storytelling can make life morally meaningful again.

It follows that if stories can provide provisional moments of reenchantment, then we need to be attentive to the sparks of spiritual impulse found in tales of lived experiences, such as this one told by a nurse at University Hospital.

I had a really difficult time accepting a family's reasoning a few years ago when they lost their two-year-old child to cancer. The way they coped/grieved was by saying that this was the way that God was testing them to see how strong they could be. I feel we are never tested in this way but this is how they were able to get through this very difficult time. I feel I should not be judgmental about how they choose to cope because I have never been put in a situation to test my ability to get through times as difficult as losing a loved one—especially a baby or child. Others have dealt with this type of situation by truly believing that their loved one is much better off and that they will eventually see them again when they "pass on" to the next life. Spirituality issues really come out when dealing with death and dying and some nurses really have the gift it takes—I am still learning how to deal with these kinds of situations and make sense of them.

As this story suggests, scientifically trained care professionals do not passively internalize transcendent understandings promoted by their organizations but must put effort into rendering them credible. One of the ways they do this is by telling stories about their experiences. But it is not simply the substance of stories that matters, but also their style. For if health professionals' stories suggest that science and spirituality are complementary, they will only be convincing (to the storytellers and perhaps their audience also) if they are composed in a way that resonates with them at a deep, subjective level. Put differently, like filmmakers, care workers will use a variety of camera lenses to lighten, color, and magnify certain features of a scene to shape how it is experienced and interpreted. This "invisible art" can make the difference between a compelling story and an ineffectual one.

This chapter analyzes nurses as storytellers: how do nurses use stories to make their daily experiences of human anguish and vulnerability spiritually meaningful? We need to pay attention to what nurses say about these experiences, but to truly appreciate the artistry that goes into retelling their encounters with illness and death, we also need to pay attention to *how* they tell their stories. What rhetorical devices or persuasive techniques do nurses use to portray spirituality in a more or less positive light? And which of these narrative tools make spirituality and science sound compatible? I explore these issues with an unexpectedly large number of stories (173) that nurses at University Hospital shared with me about work-related experiences that significantly impacted their understanding of spirituality.[1] Findings suggest that nurses compose their storied encounters with patients using a variety of rhetorical tools, but the only ones that help convince them that medical science and spirituality are compatible are those that health professionals also use when offering definitive diagnoses and describing the sacrificial nature of their work. This point suggests that fanning the embers of caritas in modern, public spaces of care will not require nurses to toss aside scientific ways of knowing but to adopt certain narrative styles found within science itself. Thus, story—the last of the five cultural mechanisms examined in this study that Weber suggested can transmit religious values—is an especially vital conduit in the work of nurses.

Some readers might prefer to go straight to the nurses' stories and skip my analysis of their rhetorical devices, just as some people prefer to experience a painting without being told by a curator about the aesthetic techniques that went into creating it. These readers can easily find the nurses' stories in block quotations. But readers interested in understanding the artistic choices involved in these rarely shared tales might indulge this curator of sorts and learn about the narrative techniques that nurses use to make spirituality come alive in a place that often censors it.

WHAT EXISTING LITERATURE SUGGESTS
ABOUT SPIRITUAL STORYTELLING

Secularization scholars have long argued that illness and other "limiting experiences" cause individuals to question spiritual understandings. From their perspective, suffering creates doubts about religious worldviews and their epistemic compatibility with science. In recent years, proponents of a lived religion perspective (Ammerman 2014; McGuire 2008) have challenged this argument. They contend that religion provides a symbolic system that enables individuals to reframe and chronicle anguishing experiences in meaningful ways as well as to create a bridge between spirituality and science. According to them, rather than constructing grand coherent theories of life or engaging in abstract debates about the compatibility of these worldviews, most people resolve such controversies through storytelling.

In focusing on individuals' experiences and how they can stamp them with spiritual meaning, the lived religion perspective also does not, as do secularization scholars, draw a sharp distinction between sacred and secular institutions. It suggests instead that individuals can carry spiritual meanings with them both inside and outside centers of worship. And unlike secularization scholars, it shifts attention away from clergy, theologians, and other religious elites, who are concerned about developing and defending coherent philosophical arguments, to nonelites, who are primarily interested in making a life (Ammerman 2006). Students of lived religion suggest that to understand how ordinary people imbue everyday life with spiritual meaning, researchers must dispense with theoretical constructs like secularization and investigate the stories that individuals tell about their experiences, including those in highly rationalized settings like the workplace.

Lived religion scholars argue that plain folks not only rely primarily on stories to make sense of their experiences, but they are especially motivated to do so when their habitual actions are unsettled by illness and other misfortunes, provoking a need for "more than ordinary" meanings. Hence, they have written extensively on how talk about health is often laced with a spiritual dimension (Ammerman 2006; McGuire 2008). Similarly, they have noted the place of spirituality in today's medical facilities, including teaching hospitals. Although these hospitals are based on the logic of bio-medicine, which has historically challenged religious understandings of suffering, academic medical centers, as pluralistic and assimilating organizations, have recently tried to bridge religious differences and acknowledge individuals' pursuit of deeper meaning by promoting a quasi-religious language of spirituality (Cadge 2013). Such language can purportedly overcome the divide between religion and science because it allows for theistic as well as nontheistic meanings (Ammerman 2013).

What makes it possible to reconcile competing outlooks is not so much the substance of spiritual stories as their style. Spirituality is a vague concept, or what linguists call a "floating signifier," which means that people can interpret it in a wide variety of ways. So whether people see spirituality and science as compatible depends on whether they speak of their spiritual lives in ways that sound consistent with naturalist norms and so seem "reasonable" (Wuthnow 2012; Evans and Evans 2008). In other words, individuals' ability to see spirituality and biomedicine as complementary depends on how well their narrative style reproduces styles typical of Western science.

Research on narrative medicine, which examines how medical care can be improved by soliciting stories from patients about their illness, likewise emphasizes the relevance of narrative and spirituality in the work of frontline health professionals (Charon 2006; see also Ten Dam and Waardenburg 2020). It argues that narratives give professionals a framework for approaching patients' problems more holistically and understanding the existential issues that often accompany illness (see also Frank 2013). It is also a method for professionals to process their experiences of caring for the sick and dying. Especially in occupations like nursing that have historical roots in religion, narrative is now being advocated as a means of self-reflection as well as a vehicle for constructing spiritual understandings (cf. Gordon 2011). In this respect, nursing differs from many other health professions that treat spirituality as being at odds with Western, rationalized medicine that emphasizes objective science (Diers 2004). A professor at University Hospital's College of Nursing, who was one of the first scholars in her discipline to champion the use of stories, said this about them: "Spirituality is a part of human nature in some way and everybody needs to discover what that part is. Stories reveal that more often than not, they bring out the depth of human nature." Her perspective echoes that of Weber, who argued that stories enable humans to make sense of their world, generate interpersonal bonds, and communicate underlying spiritual truths in ways that facts and figures cannot.

Shortcomings

Despite their interest in how stories can close the gap between religion and science, the literatures on lived religion and narrative medicine have not systematically investigated the stories of those helping professionals who care most directly for the sick and are at the forefront of the spirituality in the health care movement—nurses. On the rare occasions when lived religion scholars have examined nurses' spiritual experiences at work and their stories about them, their focus on nurses has largely been due to chance (cf. Cadge and Hammonds 2012). That is, researchers have investigated the experiences of a broad cross section of subjects, some of whom just happen to be nurses (e.g., Ammerman 2013).

Research on narrative medicine has provided numerous accounts of encounters between nurses and patients, suggesting how reflecting on such episodes can facilitate nurses' professional and personal growth (e.g., Levett-Jones 2007). But when this literature turns to the topic of spirituality, the focus is almost invariably on patients' rather than nurses' spiritual understandings (Herman 2006). Researchers, for example, stress how nurses might better understand patients' spiritual needs by giving patients the opportunity to express their experiences in the form of stories (Brody 2003). The closest these scholars come to addressing the spiritual meanings that nurses attach to their work is to examine nurses' religious and/or spiritual motivations for entering their profession (Burkhart and Hogan 2008). Because this research fails to go the next step and examine how nurses' subsequent work experiences shape their understanding of spirituality, however, it often creates the false impression that nurses compartmentalize their thoughts about work and spirituality (see Chambliss 1996).

Similarly, several nurses at University Hospital doubted that their coworkers would share stories about incidents at work that shaped their understanding of spirituality. As one nurse put it, "Most nurses are not used to talking about spirituality. They might talk about it in the classroom, but the reality is that most people don't talk about it . . . We have a lot of folklore in nursing, to be sure. But nurses are not going to share with you their folklore about spirituality." This is partly why I was surprised that nurses at University Hospital were so forthcoming in the survey about experiences at work that shaped their spirituality. Their response also suggests that despite the pluralistic ignorance surrounding spiritual talk, which we examined in a previous chapter, many nurses are quite willing to share their thoughts about spirituality if they are simply given permission to do so.

As Weber (1958c) suggests, being face-to-face with suffering can make us question our spiritual understandings and prompt us to create new ones that can speak to this suffering. And as research and lived religion and narrative medicine tell us, storytelling is one of the main ways we create new spiritual understandings. So far, this research has stopped short of examining how nurses use storytelling to develop a sacred consciousness. It doesn't tell us what kinds of rhetorical devices might enable helping professionals to reconcile rational and nonrational worldviews to cast their work-related events in a spiritual light. This is not to suggest that both literatures are uninterested in the craft of storytelling. Lived religion researchers recommend, for instance, examining commonsense narrative elements like characters, settings, props, and the sequencing of action to determine whether plots have spiritual means and ends (Ammerman 2013). But they do not get at the underlying tools that storytellers use to convince themselves and their audiences that their spiritual interpretation of an event is plausible. A story line is only compelling when told in a way that resonates with an audience, which requires the skillful application of rhetorical techniques. Likewise, suggesting that some stories go to greater lengths than others to sound reasonable begs the question of what techniques were used to achieve such an effect. In the case of nurses, then, it remains unclear which rhetorical tools they might use to imbue their work experiences with spiritual meanings and convince themselves that the gap between spiritual and scientific outlooks can be bridged.[3]

Fortunately, another set of studies, discussed in the sections that follow, suggests what those devices might be.

RHETORICAL DEVICES AND THE NARRATIVE
STYLES OF NURSES

Devout religious people sometimes don't see themselves and their world the way Western rationality would prescribe, as we know from scholarship on moral images (Greeley 1997), framing techniques (Wuthnow 1992), ethical orientations (Gilligan 1982), and modes of self-presentation (Gilligan 2003). These individuals have a certain style of describing their experiences, a particular set of interpretive lenses they employ that makes the spiritual credible to them. Western rationality depicts the sacred as absent, relies on literal language that restricts meaning, emphasizes individual rights, and discourages the expression of personal feelings. By contrast, religious people often portray the sacred as close at hand, use figurative language that expands meaning, emphasize social relationships, and acknowledge emotions. In following text, I describe these contrasting ways of portraying reality using the scholarly terms for them: *dialectical and analogical forms of imagination, centripetal and centrifugal framings, ethics of justice and care,* and *sacrificial and expressive modes of self.*

For the purposes of this study, I label these factors rhetorical devices. Rhetorical analysis, or the study of the art of persuasion, can be traced back to Aristotle, who was interested in how word choice, metaphor, and sentence structure enable orators to convince audiences that their interpretation of a situation is the correct one. These elements of style are not the same ones examined here, but those I have selected perform the same basic function, which is to persuade listeners that a storyteller's rendition of an event is credible. For that reason, I discuss the scholarly terms just mentioned as rhetorical devices. As I will show, they are some of the tools that nurses use to make the spiritual come alive or doubtful in their work and thus shape whether caritas as an experience lives on in modern care facilities.

Dialectical and Analogical Imagination

The religious imagination associated with Protestantism—and that, ironically, gave rise to modern secular thought—assumes that the divine is radically absent from the world (Greeley 1997). It pictures nature as

"God-forsaken" and society as inherently sinful and oppressive. It suggests, therefore, that the good exists apart from everyday reality. In contrast to this dialectical worldview, Greeley (1997) argues that an analogical outlook associated with religions like Catholicism assumes that the divine is manifestly present in the world. It portrays creation as a "sacrament" and society as a set of ordered relationships that, however imperfectly, reveal the value of love. Unlike its dialectical counterpart, then, this form of religious imagination suggests that the good is immanent in everyday reality, including the world of care.

Centripetal and Centrifugal Framing

The concepts of centripetal and centrifugal framing arose in literary criticism (Frye 1957) and were developed in sociology by Robert Wuthnow (1992, 2011) to describe the two main strategies people use when they talk about their experiences. On one hand, individuals who wish to suggest that an experience is subject to a single interpretation will often rely on centripetal techniques like repetition that effectively close down meaning, as is typical of Western science. On the other hand, individuals who wish to suggest that an experience is open to multiple interpretations, including spiritual ones, favor centrifugal techniques like metaphor that effectively open up meaning.

Justice and Care Ethic

The model of ethical reasoning advanced by political philosophers (e.g., Locke, Rawls, Kant) and cognitive psychologists (e.g., Kohlberg), and which informs most modern bureaucracies, is founded on the notion of justice. This orientation is concerned with substantive matters of individual rights, relies on abstract principles, emphasizes issues of independence, and justifies actions based on accepted standards and universal rules. There is, however, another orientation often glossed over by this ethic that has traditionally informed nurturant work like nursing and shapes how it is interpreted. What Gilligan (1982) labels an ethic of care is concerned with substantive matters of personal relationships and avoiding hurt to others, and it rejects abstract principles and universalist pretensions. It focuses instead on contextual detail, stresses alleviating suffering, and legitimates actions based on the special emotional, social, or spiritual needs of others.

Sacrificial and Expressive Self

People seem to experience caregiving differently depending on whether they adopt a stance that allows them to express their authentic feelings. Those who use what Gilligan (2003) calls a feminine or conventional mode of self-representation tend to sacrifice their own emotions, including spiritually tinged ones, to focus on fulfilling their roles and duties. In contrast, those who subscribe to what she calls a feminist or postconventional mode of self-representation emphasize personal authenticity. These two modes manifest themselves when caregivers give accounts of their experiences and emphasize the importance of displaying or suppressing their personal feelings.

Reflections on Rhetorical Devices

As my descriptions of these devices suggest, one of each of the pairs is more amenable than the other to the kinds of personalistic meanings that Western science denies. But that tendency isn't exclusive: people can use all eight rhetorical devices to communicate personalistic meanings. So, for example, Greeley notes that a dialectical imagination, which is associated with instrumental rationalization, is often exercised by conservative Protestants to describe a distant, spiritual dimension of reality. A conventional mode of self-expression, which stresses putting others' feelings before one's own, may be a way to revere suffering others and create space for them to share spiritual concerns. Similarly, although these pairs of devices are often presented in binary terms and studied separately, scholars recognize that each can be more or less present in a story and they can be used together. This means that storytellers might calibrate and combine different devices to achieve the rhetorical effect they're after.

The next section develops these ideas further by building on a theoretical model (Becker et al. 1976) that speaks to how health professionals construct concepts like spirituality.

HOW HELPING PROFESSIONALS CRAFT SPIRITUAL UNDERSTANDINGS

The Symbolic Interactionist Perspective on Health Care Work

Health care professions have long been a topic of study for scholars aligned with a research tradition called Chicago School symbolic interactionism (Becker et al. 1976). Scholars in this tradition describe health care work as a type of moral project. The central tenets of this perspective are that (1) people act toward things based on the meanings they ascribe to those things, (2) people learn what meanings to ascribe to things by interacting with other people, and (3) people interpret what a thing means when they're dealing with it in a specific circumstance. Viewed from the symbolic interactionists' meaning-making perspective, hospital staff act on what they believe is true, not on what is defined as true by experts (e.g., scientists, theologians). Workers, therefore, can construct understandings of things that depart from authorities' definitions. For example, whereas physicians trained in biomedicine may deny that there exists a spirit behind the body, nurses have been traditionally instructed to think the opposite. As with other types of personalistic meanings, nurses' thoughts about spirituality are not monolithic but subject to different interpretations. These interpretations are communicated and negotiated primarily, though not exclusively, through nurses' use of stories.

Extending these ideas, I argue that when describing work-related experiences, nurses and other caregivers (England 2005) can use rhetorical devices like an analogical imagination, a centrifugal frame, a care ethic, and an expressive mode of self-presentation to portray spiritual meanings as plausible even within modern hospitals whose dominant lexicon of science dismisses or discount such meanings. Nurses might, for example, use an analogical imagination to describe how belonging to a particular unit of the hospital and the bonds of friendship they experience within it make the spiritual more credible to them. It is also possible, however, that even devices that support the scientific logic of instrumental rationality and seem antithetical to the spiritual (a dialectical imagination, a centripetal frame, a justice ethic, and a sacrificial mode of self-presentation) are capable of rendering spirituality plausible. Some nurses, for instance, might use a dialectical imagination to suggest that there exist spiritual realities in the form of a faraway heaven or that patients will ultimately triumph over suffering in an afterlife. Likewise, a centripetal framing might be used by a nurse to claim in no uncertain terms that supernatural forces are real (see Wuthnow 2011).

Regardless of the type of device used, though, no device by itself is likely enough to make the spirit rationally legitimate. Usually people must combine several devices to produce an interpretation that will make spirituality sound reasonable. Caregivers can import these devices and combinations of devices into their work settings because they're readily available in the wider storytelling community outside the hospital. In other words, caregivers' choices of devices come from the larger society; these choices are not unique to them as individuals, and they don't depend purely on nurses' individual attributes, such as gender, or circumstances, such as the kinds of patients they typically care for. For example, if a nurse interprets her interactions with a dying infant through the lens of an analogical imagination that brings out the intrinsic goodness of people, it cannot be assumed that she does this simply because she is a woman who works with innocent children.

While in principle all devices can render spiritual meanings plausible, some are more stylistically congenial to the logic of instrumental rationalization than others. In particular, a dialectical imagination, a centripetal frame, a justice ethic, and a sacrificial mode of self-presentation resonate more with a Western scientific way of knowing. In fact, some symbolic interactionists have suggested that the only way to effectively question the assumptions of a scientific context and suggest, for example, that the spiritual is important is by using the devices that are typically used and considered legitimate in that context (Frank 2002). Therefore, depending on which devices caregivers rely on when reconstructing their experiences, some of them will make it easier for them to believe that medical science and spirituality are compatible.

Predictions

These ideas lead to the following testable predictions:

PREDICTION 1: When asked to describe work-related experiences of spirituality, nurses will combine rhetorical devices in multiple ways to present spirituality in a positive, plausible light.

PREDICTION 2: These combinations (or what I call narrative styles) will be independent of nurses' attributes and circumstances.

PREDICTION 3: Nurses whose narrative styles feature devices associated with instrumental reasoning will be more likely to think that spirituality and science can coexist.

METHODS

To test these predictions, I analyzed 173 stories that nurses shared in response to an open-ended survey question that asked whether they had ever had an experience at work that greatly influenced their understanding of spirituality and, if so, to describe that experience. Stories ranged from one to eleven paragraphs in length. Because I did not want nurses to feel pressure to give the "right answer" or the one they thought the researcher wanted, I chose to ask them about their experiences using an anonymous survey. The diverse responses to this survey question suggest that nurses felt comfortable telling stories that reflected their honest opinions. I also wanted to make sure that nurses who shared a story did not have significantly different opinions about spirituality than those who did not provide a story. So I compared both groups' mean answers to the survey's closed-ended questions. Their answers did not greatly differ with one important exception: those who did not report an experience were significantly less likely to agree with the statement "I am comfortable talking about spirituality." This finding suggests that nurses who provided a story had a similar perspective on spirituality to those who did not but were simply more at ease sharing their personal experiences.

To determine whether nurses portrayed spirituality positive or negatively, stories were coded using the following scheme:

1 = Positive effect (describes the spiritual as meaningful, relevant, or beneficial)

.75 = Mostly positive effect (suggests that the spiritual is largely positive but can also be ambiguous or negative)

.5 = Ambiguous effect (describes the spiritual as baffling, tangential, nebulous, or trivial)

.25 = Mostly negative effect (suggests that the spiritual is largely negative but can also be ambiguous or positive)

0 = Negative effect (describes the spiritual as pointless, irrelevant, or harmful)

To determine whether nurses think that spirituality and medicine are compatible, I used a survey question that asked nurses whether they agreed or disagreed with the statement "Promoting spirituality is at odds with the real purpose of medicine" (1 = Strongly Disagree, 2 = Disagree, 3 = Agree, 4 = Strongly Agree).

To measure the rhetorical devices, I developed a coding scheme that captures the degree to which each of the eight devices appears in a nurse's account (details about how these devices were measured, along with a discussion of my analytic strategy, can be found in the appendix to chapter 7). Scores for each device range from 1 (Fully Present) to 0 (Completely Absent).

NURSES' SPIRITUAL TALES

Table 7.1 reports that 87 percent of the stories volunteered by nurses described incidents that had a positive impact on their understanding of spirituality. Also, nurses, on average, rejected the idea that spirituality is incompatible with medicine, with their mean response (1.65) falling between Strongly Disagree (1) and Disagree (2). Of the rhetorical devices, the one most commonly used was a centripetal framing, which suggests that a reported experience is subject to a single interpretation. The least common was a justice device, which expresses a concern for matters of rights and autonomy. Table 7.1 also provides shorthand explanations of the rhetorical devices that the reader can refer to in the analyses that follow. And it reports how nurses differ in terms of gender, tenure, and spiritual or religious identities, as well as how long their typical patients stay in the hospital and their likelihood of dying. I take these factors into account when analyzing the association between rhetorical devices and whether nurses' stories portray spirituality in a positive or negative light to rule out the possibility that the rhetorical devises used by nurses are really a reflection of their personal attributes and work conditions.

Story Themes

Before the three predictions were tested, an analysis of nurses' stories and their primary themes was conducted. As table 7.2 reports, this analysis uncovered nineteen different motifs, which fell into five basic categories or

TABLE 7.1
Descriptive statistics and nurses' use of rhetorical devices in storytelling

Variable	Mean	Standard deviation	Minimum	Maximum
Outcomes				
Positive, spiritual experience at work	.87	.24	0	1
Spirituality is at odds with the purpose of medicine	1.65	.65	1	4
Rhetorical devices				
DIALECTICAL—Emphasizes how the spiritual transcends everyday reality	.37	.46	0	1
ANALOGICAL—Emphasizes how the spiritual is immanent in everyday reality	.56	.35	0	1
CENTRIPETAL—Suggests that an experience is subject to a single interpretation	.72	.39	0	1
CENTRIFUGAL—Suggests that an experience is subject to multiple interpretations	.25	.31	0	1
JUSTICE—Expresses a concern for justice, rights, and autonomy	.05	.19	0	1
CARE—Expresses a concern for personal relationships and avoiding hurt to others	.66	.30	0	1
SACRIFICIAL—Stresses the performance of roles and duties	.71	.33	0	1
EXPRESSIVE—Stresses personal authenticity	.49	.33	0	1
Other potentially relevant factors				
Years in nursing	14.81	10.04	.1	41
Gender (1 = Female)	.94	.25	0	1
Patients stay less than 1 week (1 = Yes)	.68	.47	0	1
Patients often die (1 = Yes)	.19	.39	0	1
Spiritual only (1 = Yes)	.50	.50	0	1
Religious only (1 = Yes)	.01	.08	0	1
Spiritual and religious (1 = Yes)	.45	.50	0	1
Not spiritual or religious (1 = Yes)	.05	.22	0	1

what I refer to as themes: spirituality is bound up with relationships, spirituality is revealed through events and transitions, spirituality is reflected in institutions and practices (such as those associated with organized religion), spirituality is subject to constraints and uncertainties, and spirituality is disappointing and baseless. These themes capture the substance (as opposed to the style) of nurses' stories.

TABLE 7.2
Primary themes of nurses' stories

Themes and motifs	Percent
Spirituality is bound up with relationships	
Comforting others makes the spiritual real	27
Suffering people can teach us spiritual lessons	9
Spirituality is mutually beneficial	3
Accepting and forgiving others require spiritual strength	2
Total	41
Spirituality is revealed through events and transitions	
Bizarre happenings speak to a higher power	9
Death is a spiritual moment	8
Birth is a spiritual moment	2
When patients need spirituality most	1
Mundane happenings speak to a higher power	1
Total	21
Spirituality is reflected in institutions and practices	
Efficacious spiritual techniques and outlooks	16
Admirable spiritual traditions and representatives	4
Total	20
Spirituality is subject to constraints and uncertainties	
Spirituality is inexplicable	5
Modern medicine dehumanizes the caring encounter	3
Patients and families respond differently to spirituality	2
Questions exist about what constitutes spirituality	2
Spirituality is found outside work	1
Total	13
Spirituality is disappointing and baseless	
Religion should have no place in health care	3
Some deaths are difficult and senseless	2
There is evil in the world	1
Total	6
	100

Stories that address the first three themes cast spirituality in the most positive terms. For example, most nurses who described spirituality as being bound up with relationships wrote of how the act of comforting others made the spiritual more real:

> One time at work years ago, I went down to the cafeteria and was waiting on the elevator to go back up to my floor. Something inside gave me the inclination to take the stairs instead. On the way up the stairs, a woman was crying very hard and leaning against the wall. I stopped and asked if I could help. She said her child was in peds ICU [pediatric intensive care unit] and not doing well at all and may die. I had no knowledge of this patient or situation. I just stayed with the mother for a few minutes . . . and prayed silently to myself for her and her child. Then I said to "keep having faith because God was with her always." She said thank you so much for talking with her and she felt better. I truly believe that God wanted me to be there at that particular time to meet that mother's needs. That incident also led me to pray for that unknown patient and to pray more to God for all my patients and other patients.
>
> I was asked to help "hold down" a geriatric patient. When I held her wrists she cried, screamed, and struggled—When I took her hands I "saw" her holding her father's hand as a child, her husband's hand through time and her children's hands—as if I became her—and she stopped struggling.

Nurses who suggested that spirituality is revealed through particular events and transitions often wrote about experiences like the following, where a bizarre occurrence convinced them of the existence of a higher power or how being with a dying patient moved them at a deep, spiritual level:

> We used to have a small trauma resuscitation room. Occasionally when cleaning up after a patient's untimely death their spirit would remain in the room. You knew they were there because there was a pocket of cold air usually near the head of the bed. I can remember one night standing in the middle of this cold air and explaining to this spirit we'd done all that we could, it was time to move on. Briefly it got colder and then warmed up. To me this power of human connection—either alive or dead is powerful—is the perfect example of spirituality.
>
> When I was in my first year of nursing I cared for a dying AIDs patient who was estranged from his father. I knew the young man would not live

long so I called his father, let him know of his son's condition, then put his son on the phone. He was somewhat confused but there was no mistaking the light in his eyes when he heard his dad's voice. The patient couldn't talk long but I did tell him to tell his dad "I love you" which he did. The patient died before the father got to the hospital, he stayed at the airport and left as soon as he could get back to his home. I knew then that this job would be VERY difficult and extremely rewarding.

Nurses who equated spirituality with particular religious institutions and practices also described very positive experiences. Most wrote about efficacious spiritual techniques and outlooks, as in this story:

I took care of a young man from Asia with leukemia who was going under bone marrow transplant from an unrelated donor. Four weeks after the transplant the team ran out of ideas and there was nothing they said they could do to improve his status. He was getting sicker and like most of the other kids on the transplant unit was fixing to die. One day I saw four monks (Buddhist) in brown garments come to see and pray for the young man . . . Within two days after the visit by the monks, the patient's condition improved 100 percent and he went home after ten days . . . I believe that the visit by the monks changed that kid's life, saved his life.

Other nurses described experiences that had an ambiguous or negative effect on their understanding of spirituality. For example, of those who suggested that spirituality is subject to constraints and uncertainties, some, like this nurse, emphasized its inexplicable nature:

A few years ago, a four-year-old boy was dying from leukemia. Although sedated the night of his demise, at [4 A.M.], with his father at his bedside he sat upright. His father said "Ryan, what's the matter?" Ryan replied, "I'm scared." His father said, "It's okay, what's scary?" Ryan then replied, "The train is going to take me." After clarification, the dad felt the train was a bright light and asked Ryan "is anyone there?" Ryan said "grandpa." Dad told Ryan to "take grandpa's hand and it would be OK." Shortly thereafter Ryan passed away—calmly and without further meds. This night will always make me wonder if there is an afterlife.

And those who suggested that spirituality is essentially baseless and disappointing often wrote of how religion has no place in health care or how senseless and difficult deaths caused them to doubt the relevance of the spiritual, or even be suspicious of others' spirituality, as illustrated in this account:

> During my fourteen years in pediatrics, I've seen too many beautiful children die to take religion or spirituality seriously.
>
> I have seen some coworkers who use the guise of "spirituality" to take advantage of people who are desperate for any sign of positive feedback to what is usually a devastating or life-threatening event in their life. So-called "spiritual" health care workers . . . really feed their own egos and reinforce to themselves what their spiritual needs may be. It quite often has nothing to do with the patient's situation . . . It is NEVER [respondent emphasis] right to inflict one's own belief system off on someone else. It lacks a subtle understanding of the human spirit.

Of the five basic types of stories told by nurses, those suggesting that spirituality is bound up with relationships were the most common (41 percent). And of the nineteen primary motifs, those suggesting that comforting others made the spiritual more real were the most frequent—over a quarter (27 percent) of nurses wrote about this particular motif. The tremendous variety in nurses' motifs speaks to how they creatively interpret and negotiate meanings like spirituality. Despite this variety, I found that nurses commonly used a few particular combinations of rhetorical devices to describe spirituality in either positive or negative terms.

Combinations of Rhetorical Devices

So, what are the devices that nurses, as storytellers, use to stylize the spiritual as more or less plausible in their accounts of work-related experiences? The answer to this question is critical to our understanding of the fate of caritas because narrative is one of the cultural mechanisms that Weber suggested can transmit religious ideals. Table 7.3 summarizes the results of an analysis of the most common ways that nurses narrate their work-related experiences in a positive, spiritual light. Devices in uppercase are those strongly present in a story, while those in lowercase are largely absent. Shorthand explanations of the rhetorical devices can be found in table 7.1.

TABLE 7.3
Narratives styles and their motifs

Narrative styles	Motifs
1. CENTRIPETAL* SACRIFICIAL* expressive	**Suffering people can teach us spiritual lessons**
2. justice*CARE*SACRIFICIAL* **CENTRIPETAL**	**Comforting others makes the spiritual real**
3. justice*EXPRESSIVE*ANALOGICAL* CENTRIPETAL	Comforting others makes the spiritual real
4. justice*CARE*ANALOGICAL* CENTRIFUGAL	Comforting others makes the spiritual real
5. CENTRIPETAL* SACRIFICIAL* dialectical	**Comforting others makes the spiritual real**

Note: The narrative styles cast nurses' storied experiences in a positive, spiritual light even after controlling for nurses' tenure, gender, the types of patients they care for, and nurses' spiritual or religious identities. Nurses who use the first, second, and fifth narrative styles (shown in bold type) are significantly more likely to disagree with the statement "Promoting spirituality is at odds with the real purpose of medicine."

Consistent with the first prediction, findings reveal that nurses combine rhetorical devices to cast the spiritual in a positive, plausible light. The first of these narrative styles, for example, uses a centripetal frame (CENTRIPETAL) that suggests that an experience is subject to a single interpretation and a sacrificial mode of self-presentation (SACRIFICIAL) that stresses the performance of roles and duties, while also refraining from using an expressive mode (expressive) that emphasizes personal authenticity.[3] Nurses who adopted this narrative style often told a story whose motif was about how suffering people can teach us spiritual lessons. The following account is an example.

I was working in an ICU unit caring for an elderly gentleman who was very ill. At the change of shift, he began to code, we began the life-saving measures we had been trained in. Shortly after, his wife entered the room and politely asked us to stop. She said "he does not want this, he has said his goodbyes and is ready to be with God." We stopped our efforts and he passed shortly after. She thanked us for our efforts and asked us for some time with him. She emerged about an hour later with a smile on her face. I asked her if she needed anything and if she was alright. She nodded and said that he is in a much better place, he's with the Lord and he has waited his whole life for this opportunity, and then she walked out of the unit. Her faith and strength in the knowledge that her loved one of 57 years was with God was amazing.

In contrast, nurses who employed the next four styles most often shared accounts of how comforting others made the spiritual real for them. Their stories speak to how the same spiritual theme can be rendered in multiple ways. The following three examples illustrate this point.

Style 2 suggests that one way nurses portray comforting others in a positive spiritual light is to show that abstract principles of justice are less important (justice) than a commitment to individualized care (CARE) and performing job responsibilities (SACRIFICIAL). In addition, they use a centripetal discursive device (CENTRIPETAL), which produces a single interpretation of an event. For example, one nurse wrote:

> While often it is a nurse's job to help a patient recover, sometimes it is our job to help them die with comfort and dignity. Once, I had a dying patient who had been very religious and spiritual during her life and had a deep faith in God. She had been almost non-responsive for a few days as her family and friends stayed close at her bedside. At one point during the afternoon, the patient's breathing became a little more labored and she seemed a little agitated. Her family and friends gathered around her and began to sing "Amazing Grace," her favorite hymn. During the second verse, she smiled a last time and died peacefully. I believe spirituality and a belief in God helped this patient to die peacefully, and helped her family and friends deal with her death. Like them, I believe she waits for them in heaven.

By defining a nurse's job in the first sentence, this story clearly emphasizes the roles and responsibilities of nursing. This story shows a commitment to personalized care, especially as the nurse takes note of the patient's favorite hymn. The story closes by attributing the peaceful death to the patient's belief in God, suggesting that the nurse concurs, thus closing off alternative interpretations.

In other examples, nurses avoid abstraction but focus on what they learned from the encounter, sometimes even telling stories of everyday life infused with spirituality, as is seen in narrative style 3 and the following example.

> I had a good friend who was dying with cancer, her husband left her and she was very alone in a crisis she could not recover from. I visited with her as often as I could and listened to her stories of her life, good, bad, and

indifferent. She was very intelligent but often misunderstood. Being there for her was important to me and her. She made an impact on my life . . . I learned to understand how just being there meant a lot to someone in great pain.

In this example, this nurse closes down meaning of the event (CENTRIP-ETAL), claiming that the encounter was good for everyone involved. But unlike in the first example, this nurse emphasizes her personal growth, showing a commitment to an expressive framing of care (EXPRESSIVE). This story also shows the ways that personal relationships—the sharing of stories and time—can be infused with spirituality (ANALOGICAL).

In a minority of cases, nurses invoked the same theme but emphasized that the interpretation of the event was open to many meanings (CEN-TRIFUGAL). Illustrating narrative style 4, the following example shows how care (CARE) and an analogical spiritual imagination (ANALOGI-CAL) can lead one to wonder about unknown spiritual matters.

Several years ago a family asked me to pray with them along with their minister and the attending physician. Their young son was critically injured in a car accident. Unfortunately, the child died several days later in the intensive care unit, but one could definitely feel the power of prayer in the room. There was an amazing sense of peace despite this tragedy that the family was enduring. The family wrote me a couple months later, saying how they were coping and adapting to the loss of their child. It was an amazing and touching letter.

The nurse mentions a "power of prayer in the room" but does not explain from where this power derived and does not provide the reader with an explicit definition of the encounter.

All of these examples highlight the importance of relationships in constructing spirituality as consistent with the administration of care. Comforting others allowed nurses to perform their official duties in personalized ways, sometimes helped nurses to learn about themselves, and showed how the everyday work of care can be infused with spirituality. These examples also speak to the effort that nurses put into making work-related experiences spiritually significant or insignificant through the deployment of various rhetorical devices.

Ruling Out the Possibility That Narrative Styles Are Simply a Reflection of the Storytellers' Attributes and Circumstances

Do nurses' narrative strategies depend on their individual attributes and circumstances? The strategies employed by nurses, for example, could be a function of their gender, number of years as a nurse, religious or spiritual identities, and whether they work with patients who are likely to die or are hospitalized long enough for nurses to get to know them. While some of these factors were found to cause nurses to translate their experiences in more positive spiritual terms—being a female, being religious and spiritual, being spiritual only, caring for patients who often die, and caring for patients who typically stay longer than a week (as the note in table 7.3 reports)—none can completely explain the observed effects of nurses' narrative styles 1 through 5. Hence, findings support the second prediction that rhetorical devices act independently of caregivers' individual attributes and circumstances.

The Compatibility of Spirituality and Medical Science

As table 7.3 also shows (see narrative styles in bold type), nurses who adopt the first narrative style to describe how suffering people can teach us spiritual lessons are significantly more likely to disagree with the notion that spirituality and medicine are at cross-purposes. The same is true of nurses who use the second and fifth styles to describe how comforting others makes the spiritual real. In contrast, those who employ the third and fourth narrative styles to describe how comforting others makes the spiritual real are no more likely to disagree with this notion than other nurses.

So, what might explain these differences? In particular, how is it possible that nurses who converge on the same theme differ over the compatibility of spirituality and medicine? The answers to these questions lie in the rhetorical devices shared by nurses who exhibit the first, second, and fifth narrative styles. Each of these strategies involves two devices—a centripetal frame and a sacrificial mode of self-expression—and thus is a variation on this basic narrative approach. Moreover, these two ways of casting lived experience are ones promoted by medical bureaucracies that stress the importance of providing definitive answers and fulfilling role obligations.

This finding comports with the third prediction that care workers who display instrumental reasoning are more likely to perceive that spiritual and biomedical orientations are compatible. It also suggests that to reduce the dissonance between these two orientations, workers must make certain concessions and adopt some of the rhetorical devices associated with modern medicine. This adjustment enables them to have two parallel sets of "right answers or interpretations."

From the perspective of knowledge experts, science and religion may seem incompatible—but ordinary people are able to fit them together. For the nurses I studied, the most common way they fit them together was by accepting conventional, biomedical understandings of their work and then using stories to add spiritual meanings to those understandings. Integrating spirituality in this way does not require nurses to argue against scientific ways of knowing; it only requires them to adopt certain narrative styles.

CONCLUSION

Despite working in seemingly unreceptive, scientific settings, nurses as storytellers are able to develop spiritual understandings of their work experiences and thus sustain the ethic of caritas. By using and combining a variety of rhetorical devices, they stylize the concept of spirituality so as to make it plausible. Contrary to the conventional wisdom that there is an irreconcilable conflict between spirituality and the medical that forces health professionals to compartmentalize the two, many hospital nurses creatively mix moral images and modes of self-presentation to depict spirituality as a credible facet of human experience. And nurses use some of these rhetorical devices to portray spirituality and medicine as complementary; that is, they use devices also used by medical staff when making definitive diagnoses and describing the sacrificial nature of their work. Hence, the moral legitimacy of hospitals hinges not so much on administrators' public acknowledgment of humanistic ideals like spirituality (Greenwood et al. 2007) as on how rank-and-file personnel artfully construct those ideals based on their interactions with patients and coworkers.

Although this study sheds new light on the power of stories to sustain caritas in clinical settings, objections about it might be raised. Some may argue that stories involving meanings like spirituality can be highly superficial and idiosyncratic. Others might fault this study because it cannot be easily replicated and generalized to other settings. Finally, some might object that in focusing on the meanings of nurses' work, it has neglected larger issues of power such as the tremendous influence exerted by Big Pharma and private insurers (see also Gordon 2011).

However, far from finding that accounts about spiritual experiences lack depth and are plagued by peculiarities, this analysis discovered that nurses often wrote about matters of life and death and that their narratives were constructed in patterned ways around recurrent themes. Granted that the experiences analyzed in this case study may not be representative of those in other nursing staffs, knowing some of the ways that caregivers construct and understand their lived experiences is as scientifically important as determining how frequently those experiences occur. Finally, although this study of hospital nurses did not do justice to the powerful actors within the health care industry, it did focus on the care providers who work directly with some of society's most vulnerable members and the health conse-quences of power imbalances.[4]

Many scholars have assumed that a type of warfare exists between reli-gion and science (for a discussion of this literature, see Evans and Evans 2008), predicting that the latter will eventually triumph over the former as modern individuals seek out more rational explanations of suffering. Considerable research on the topic, therefore, has focused on the changing status of religious and scientific experts and the clash between the precisely argued philosophical systems they proffer. But my findings suggest that rational argument is only one way, and certainly not the best way, of navi-gating between these two systems. Ordinary people who aren't religious or scientific experts may not think about the relationship between religion and science in terms of which has the better arguments. Instead, they may think of this relationship in more pragmatic terms, especially when tend-ing to the needs of vulnerable others. In that case, "hybridizers," or workers who can simultaneously embrace two competing logics like medicine and spirituality, may be in a particularly favorable position not only to lead modern organizations through adaptation and innovation (see Pache and Santos 2013) but also preserve the religious ethic of caritas.

Still, if current debates are any indication, many intellectuals will con-tinue to assume that the answer to societal challenges ultimately depends on experts like themselves who are trained to devise cognitive fixes. And yet, judging from my postsurgery experiences at least, purely intellectual attempts to reconcile spirituality and science seem vain. To truly reconcile these competing systems of value, we need to be able to engage with vulnerable strangers as human beings, not just talk about them as hypothetical abstractions. In the end, where spirituality and science may come together is in the experience of care.

Two days after I visit my dad, I'm awakened at night by a medical social worker who tells me that I'll be discharged in the morning. After I gather my clothes and other belongings, I visit my dad one last time to let him know that I'll be waiting for him in Arizona. Dr. Marcos and his team won't be returning to the floor until after I'm discharged, so I ask the social worker to thank them for all they've done for us. In the morning, my wife takes our three daughters and me to the Pittsburgh International Airport for a flight back to Tucson. I follow her harried lead to a cab, bent over and watching each step I take to prevent a fall. At the airport, the security officers tell me I can't rest in a wheelchair but must stand in line to be checked in. As we wait behind an endless line of college students returning to school, I can barely maintain an upright position and must occasionally crouch to rest and regain my strength.

When I finally arrive home, I insist on pulling myself up the banister to our upstairs bedroom. Before collapsing on the bed, I pause and view my stomach in the wall mirror above the dresser. I touch a swollen section of the incision and discover two silver staples the surgical team apparently forgot about, which explains why I set off an alarm earlier when entering and exiting the hospital's gift shop. I have them removed by my family physician two days later.

My department head generously offers to give me time off to recover from the surgery, but I decline, not wanting to fall behind in my work. The day before classes start, I hobble across campus to my office. Looking out its window to the north, I see the hospital where I had interned as a chaplain. To the west, the late afternoon sun begins to drop behind the Tucson Mountains, casting a shadow on the city below that stretches unevenly beyond buildings of various heights.

Later, as I trudge back to my car, I am intercepted by a student wanting to be added to my already full class on social problems. He goes on about his desperate need to be enrolled, hinting that I owe him a favor, that I, and I alone, stand between this "lifelong Arizona resident" and his graduation. As he holds out an add-form for me to sign, I can't help but notice his resolute posture, his head up, his shoulders back, and his legs in an upside-down V that positions him solidly on the burnt grass. Having just come home feeling physically, emotionally, and spiritually drained, his demanding attitude just reinforces my sense of emptiness.

The whistle of the Union Pacific Railroad that runs from Nogales to Tucson sounds in the distance. Looking over the shoulder of the student and in the direction of the train, I recall the surgeons scrambling to graft the truncated leg of an undocumented worker. I then imagine that same immigrant staggering through the Sonoran Desert's deadly heat. He emerges from its blinding, shimmering mirages, only to discover that the passage from an enchanted world to a supposedly enlightened one is neither fair nor seamless. Like foreign tissue transplanted into an ailing, dispirited host, he is mistakenly rejected as a threat.

It is a story and vision I would like to share with this anxious undergrad, who has now positioned himself so that his eyes look directly into mine. But I suspect that the spiritual issues the experience raised for me about the perilous state of being a human would probably be lost on him unless he had personally tended to someone involved in a similar tragedy. And so, like a lot of nurses, I keep this spiritual tale to myself.

Chapter Eight

RESTORING THE SANCTITY ONCE
BESTOWED ON HUMANITY

Can humanity restore the sanctity that religion once bestowed upon it while continuing to reap the benefits of rationalization? The answer to that question, Weber suggested, will decide the fate of caritas, the Axial principle that benevolence must be extended to all, including strangers, because all humans possess a transcendent dignity at the center of their personhood. As I have discussed it here, caritas goes beyond feeling sorry for vulnerable others or tending to their physical or emotional state by also acknowledging them as spiritual beings. It thus addresses the horizontal dimension of religion, which asserts that the sacred resides in us (as opposed to a distant, supernatural realm), and, in that sense, is consistent with humanistic conceptions of individuals as inherently good. Today, this ethic often goes by the name of spiritual care and is considered to be one facet of a holistic or person-centered approach to well-being.

According to Weber, caritas can establish a niche in secular settings to the extent that actors within them assume responsibility for spiritual care, talk about spirituality among themselves, can believe that their work has spiritual import without feeling disingenuous, practice spiritual care, and reconcile the tensions between rationality and spirituality through stories about their lived experiences. While some of these mechanisms, such as taking over for spiritual care and performing acts that address others' spiritual needs, most obviously manifest the ethic of caritas, that ethic also needs to be realized through the other mechanisms to seem credible and be institutionalized. To advance our understanding of this ethic's status in contemporary society, this book examined how an academic medical center's nursing staff negotiated spirituality through these mechanisms. And to further illuminate the need for caritas and the tensions involved in integrating it into a rationalized setting, I described my experiences as a chaplain intern and as a living liver transplant donor at two teaching hospitals.

While preparing my study, I came across an administrator in University Hospital's patient services division who seemed extremely knowledgeable about the Axial principle of caritas. When asked in a presurvey interview what place spirituality had in nursing, she answered,

> I think nurses should take care of people like you would take care of your mom or dad, or brothers and sisters. You may not like them, but they deserve the best. Whatever resentments, etc. you might have about a patient, when you hit that door, you should leave them behind . . . That is why it is so important to view patients through a spiritual lens. . . . To be spiritual, doesn't mean you have to be a Christian. You could be Muslim, for example. Islam says you have to be permissive of other religions and so it doesn't necessarily consider Christianity or Buddhism as bad. The gods of the Greeks inspired a similar outlook . . . As long as you believe in something, as long as you've lived life to the best, you have fulfilled the golden rule. It is in every single religion, in every single spirituality.

While her response suggested that caritas as an idea was alive and well at her hospital, survey results confirmed my hunch that integrating this ethic into nurses' science-based care was more complicated and not readily apparent. As discussed in chapter 3, after learning that University Hospital planned to terminate its entire chaplaincy program, nearly a third of nurses said they would be willing to step in for chaplains and take on responsibility for patients' spiritual care. Indeed, an even larger percentage claimed they already provided more spiritual care than chaplains. This response suggested that if conventional religious figures were eliminated, religious authority could still be transferred to others.

Although many nurses were open to performing clergy-like roles, however, chapter 4 revealed that they rarely talked about spiritual matters among themselves. A large majority (85 percent) said they were quite comfortable discussing spiritual matters but they also were under the false impression that this was not the case with most of their peers. Hence, a veil of pluralistic ignorance prevented nurses from broaching the topic of spirituality at official gatherings. Also stopping spirituality from sticking at University Hospital was the fact that it did not emotionally resonate with all nurses. Many nurses, in fact, were torn about describing their science-based care as spiritually significant, as discussed in chapter 5. Factors at work and elsewhere that convinced some nurses that there was something spiritual about their care work also enabled them to feel that their work was an extension of their true selves. But for others, what led them to believe their work was spiritual put pressure on them to suppress their true feelings. Working with seriously ill patients, for example, sensitized some nurses to spiritual issues and led them to acknowledge the place of spirituality in their work, but working with those same types of patients also put a limit on the emotions they could express.

Despite these communication barriers and emotional risks, chapter 6 showed that a significant minority of nurses who view their work in spiritual terms as a type of calling systematically applied a variety of spiritual therapies in a variety of situations. These "internal activists" were instrumental in translating their hospital's advertised commitment to spiritual care into subtle but tangible deeds. And contrary to the idea that ordinary people choose between the arguments of religious and scientific experts, chapter 7 uncovered how most nurses adjudicate these perspectives through stories about experiences with patients. These rarely shared tales were often crafted in ways that not only made the spiritual plausible but also suggested how science and spirituality can coexist.

Spirituality's place in the halls of medicine was not immediately obvious to me as a participant, either. In fact, if I had judged solely from my experience as a liver donor, I might have concluded that the ethic of caritas had been entirely hollowed out from the transplant center. And yet, having previously spent time as a chaplain intern and relied so heavily on nurses' advice about how to address patients' spiritual needs, I knew that the promise made by two nurses to be with my dad and me should the transplant procedure fail was more than idle talk. It was code for a commitment to valuing patients as persons or, in our case, treating us as more than organs and arteries.

So, what do these findings suggest about the status of caritas? Contrary to those who suggest that its fate depends on leaders adopting an Axial mindset (Barnes 2009; Baskin and Bondarenko 2014; Tang 2016), results indicate that it hinges more on the five cultural mechanisms identified by Weber for transmitting ideals—authority, language, emotions, actions, and narrative—and whether they are enabled at the level where care is actually delivered. If caritas, to use Weber's famous phrase, is to avoid becoming another "ghost of dead beliefs," it must stick through these channels. The fact that some of these channels—language and emotions—were problematic speaks to the unstable, fragile nature of caritas. Then again, the fact that the others—authority, actions, and narrative—were at least partially effective suggests how caritas can still establish a toehold in secularized settings.

As demonstrated here, teaching hospitals provide a great window into the survival of caritas because they are so hemmed in by not only science but also public funding and bureaucracy. This situation sheds light on spirituality in a rationalized setting more broadly, both the challenges and possibilities. On the other hand, when we step back and look at society as a whole, we notice that not every setting is so hemmed in by rationalization. There are subaltern pockets and spaces outside the conventional medical system like public schools, community counseling centers, social work agencies, and fire stations where holistic care may flourish in a kind of dance with the dominant force of rationalization. The fate of caritas is being decided in these types of settings as well.

Results also underscore the importance of actors other than traditional religious authorities in determining the survival of this ethic. As moral placeholders of sorts, frontline helping professionals play a pivotal role in integrating caritas in the public sphere. Far from being neutral messengers of institutions who merely follow the ideological lead of their superiors, these workers must actively negotiate corporate-sponsored meanings like spirituality in their interactions with vulnerable strangers lest their organizations be accused of only paying lip service to the public's ideals.

In addition to pinch-hitting for religious figures, these workers often function as stand-ins for friends and family who affirm the vulnerable person's intrinsic worth. One nurse spoke to this role played by care workers when she said,

A patient's daughter was a scientist in northeast Africa and was flying here to be with her mom before she passed. She did not make it in time. Her mom died about half an hour before her arrival. Two months later I received a letter from the daughter, thanking me for holding her hand and talking to her up to the time of her passing . . . I adored and cherished my grandparents. They are both gone, but I remembered what it was like to have them here and so when the daughter said thank you for being with her mom and for helping her, I knew . . . yeah this is great . . . being a nurse has definitely got to be the most stressful and the most rewarding job at the same time. And spirituality has to enter it, because if you don't have it, you and your patient are going to lose it.

Importantly, the sacred texts of many world religions mention a similar bridging role. In Christianity, for example, believers are told: "You are the salt of the earth" (Matthew 5:13). The phrase means that followers are expected neither to dominate the world nor retreat from it. Instead, it urges individuals to find a middle path of service and compassion (Ricoeur 1958). Even though that path may be difficult to discern or chart, only by following it can religion be the salt that transforms society.

Nurses tread one such interstitial pathway. Where it will lead in the coming years is uncertain, but it could be consequential in the wake of the precipitous decline in religiosity. In a paper titled "Giving Up on God," Ronald Inglehart (2020) reports that from 2007 to 2019, the vast majority of the countries he studied—43 out of 49—became less religious. The decline in belief was not limited to high-income countries but appeared across most of the world. Nurses might accelerate this trend by resisting pressure to acknowledge and address the afflicted as whole persons with spiritual needs. Or, as care workers on the "edge of religion," they might continue to engage spirituality and act as surrogates of religious authorities during these lean years. Either way, nurses will likely play an important role in deciding the fate of religion's chief social contribution—the Axial ethic that all vulnerable strangers have infinite value and are deserving of care. Indeed, during a time when many are turning away from religion, the small number of helping professionals who remain committed to caritas may function as an "abeyance structure" (Taylor 1989) that holds and sustains the two-thousand-year-old caritas movement as it moves from one stage of history to the next.

Nurses may suspend caritas long enough for organized religion to recover and become again the source and sustenance of this ethic. But they and other care workers might also help to sustain caritas more widely. That is, in addition to organized religion, caritas could be sustained by more secular forces—humanism, political movements, and psychotherapeutic models. In fact, in suggesting that religion was no longer strong enough to preserve caritas but that it could still be transmitted through various cultural mechanisms, Weber pointed to the possibility that there might be alternative supports for the ethic. As actors at the intersection of the secular and sacred, frontline care workers like nurses could play a decisive part in strengthening or weakening such props.

A NEW WAY OF THINKING ABOUT RELIGION IN THE PUBLIC SQUARE

This book's attention to frontline helping professionals points to a new understanding of spirituality in secular institutions that complements the two leading academic perspectives on public religion. The dominant secularization perspective, which is commonly thought to be the one Weber expressed, suggests that modern individuals can only acquire a fragmented and idiosyncratic sense of sacredness. According to proponents of this view (e.g., Norris and Inglehart 2004), rationalization pressures religion to fashion more coherent doctrines than the ones it has traditionally offered to explain the phenomenon of "undeserved suffering" (see Weber 1958d). At the same time, rationalization spurs other "value spheres"—the economy, the state, education, art, and intimate relationships—that develop their own distinct logics. Rationalization thus challenges and circumscribes the views of religious authorities, and in doing so, it shifts responsibility for moral decision-making from religious communities to individuals, who are freed to develop their own worldviews. As a result of these processes of differentiation and individuation, religion is reduced from a "sacred canopy" that gives every dimension of life moral meaning to just one of several institutions competing for individuals' allegiance. And this decline of religious meaning leads humanity to think of itself in increasingly secular and subjective terms. Nonreligious institutions such as scientific hospitals may occasionally accommodate traditional religious beliefs, but they'll do so in superficial or cynical ways, because these institutions' truth claims are fundamentally at odds with those of religion. In short, from a secularization perspective, the sacred canopy of religion that had recognized humans as spiritual beings will be gradually reduced, disfigured, and cast aside.

Scholars who subscribe to a lived religion perspective, inspired by Durkheim (Seidman 1985), reject the secularization thesis and suggest that humanity's sanctity will remain intact and even be deepened. They argue that every society rests on a religiously based set of shared moral understandings that integrate personal and social systems, though the form of religious life varies over time. Differentiation, from this perspective, doesn't isolate religion; instead it breaks monopolistic religions down into diverse, decentralized, and voluntary moral communities that crystallize the common life of their members. And individuation, instead of freeing individuals from the sacred, infuses ordinary existence with transcendent meaning and makes the divine more immanent by making the self the sacred, unifying object of society. When religion is no longer enforced from above, people's spiritual or "more than ordinary" experiences fill them with enthusiasm from below (Joas 2013). While naturalist worldviews may threaten the plausibility of such transcendent understandings, they rarely cause people to experience cognitive dissonance, because most avoid making claims that violate commonsense norms of reasonableness (Wuthnow 2012). More generally, the lived religion perspective contends that modern individuals can still experience a sense of spiritual wholeness by drawing on the support of their chosen "spiritual tribes" (Ammerman 2014)—close-knit groups operating within or outside of organized religion that invent, develop, and adapt cultural resources to invoke the sacred in everyday life.

Both perspectives have advanced our understanding of rationalization and the problem of meaning. But both also mischaracterize Weber as a cultural pessimist (Seidman 1985) and, more importantly, stop short of addressing what most concerned him about rationalization—the possibility that it would expel religion's ethic of caritas (care) from public life (Kalberg 1990; Bellah 1999; Symonds and Pudsey 2006; Symonds 2016). Weber certainly described rationalization in bleak terms and spoke of science as a "specifically irreligious power." But he also thought that the religious ethic of caritas would continue to be the ideal against which other, less personal value spheres would be judged. He believed that the unexpected harm caused by bureaucracies and technology could paradoxically increase charismatic needs and stimulate a desire to rehumanize relationships in ways consistent with caritas. And he implicitly recommended caritas to people who worked in scientific environments as a way to stay sensitive to others' suffering.

When I say that secularization scholars and their critics have neglected caritas, I don't mean that they're uninterested in care and the plight of the vulnerable. Both camps suggest that transformations of religion, whether in the guise of a new theodicy or human rights policy, stem from a desire to lessen human suffering. Secularization researchers have addressed care by studying leaders and experts who are responsible for identifying needs in the wider society and enlisting others to meet them (Chaves 1994). And lived religion scholars have addressed spirituality and the alleviation of suffering by studying people who rely on spirituality as a source of personal healing (McGuire 2008; Ammerman 2014).

Neither group, however, examines professional care workers—people who are paid to care for the well-being of others or engage in hands-on, "interactive care work" (Folbre 2012). The scientists, theologians, and other authority figures studied by secularization researchers typically occupy powerful positions that are far removed from the face-to-face delivery of care (Tronto 1993; see also Glenn 2012). And the afflicted individuals examined by lived religion scholars are focused on self-care, not care of others. On the rare occasions that these two sets of scholars have investigated people who directly care for others, they have focused on volunteers (Wuthnow 2012) or members of congregations who just happen to be helping professionals (Ammerman 2014). As these researchers note (e.g., Ammerman 1997), the circle of care even among so-called Golden Rule Christians tends to be narrow, confined to family, friends, neighbors, and congregations, in what Stephen Warner (1988) refers to as "elective parochialism"; see also Tronto's (2013, 13–14) discussion of the dangers of parochialism within care.

As institutions become more and more rationalized, hospitals and other modern care facilities are increasingly held accountable for rationalization's dehumanizing effects. Patient satisfaction surveys, for example, define good outcomes in terms of what is meaningful and valuable to the individual patient (see Bromley and Powell 2012), and, in response, hospitals have begun promoting humanistic values like spirituality (see Cadge 2013). Consequently, their frontline care workers are now expected to fashion moral orders that accommodate multiple spiritual tribes while still operating under an instrumental rationality that is indifferent if not hostile to such nonmaterialist orientations.

When we focus on professional care workers, we see people trying to integrate caritas into a rationalized setting in their daily lives at work. We

TABLE 8.1

Comparison of secularization, lived religion, and caritas perspectives

	Secularization	Lived religion	Caritas
Chief actors	Religious and secular elite	Ordinary people	Caregivers
Defining problem	Conflicting truth claims and boundary maintenance	Making a life	Loss of the human
Conception of rationalization	Steel shell or iron cage	Pliable shell or cage	Sintered shell or cage
Characterization of religion	Distinct beliefs and value sphere	Portable experiences	Person-giving relationships

see the concrete challenges of this project and the solutions that may be possible. What's more, a focus on caring professionals can complement the secularization and lived religion perspectives in shining a light on facets of public religion that their frameworks do not address. I sketch the contours of this caritas framework in table 8.1. To understand how this framework adds to the two dominant perspectives on modern religion, I compare the caritas perspective to the other two perspectives along four key dimensions: whom they treat as the chief actors, what they consider to be the defining problem, their conceptions of rationalization, and their characterizations of religion.

Chief Actors

The secularization perspective concentrates on leaders of epistemic movements, cultural trendsetters, institutional gatekeepers, and others who control vast resources and have a decidedly strong religious or scientific orientation. The lived religion approach focuses on individuals whose quotidian existence is either grounded in religious institutions that prescribe traditional rituals or in spaces outside them that are not subject to religious authorities but where individuals innovate spiritual habits for themselves. In contrast, a caritas approach casts its analytical lens on those who protect and nurture vulnerable people. In the past, these actors consisted exclusively of friends, family, and other intimates. Today they are increasingly helping professionals from the public sector who are expected to translate, negotiate, and instantiate society's humanistic ideals. These actors inhabit local worlds, such as health care organizations, where the tensions between religion and science are especially acute, inviting scrutiny of their understandings of suffering and the moral authority of their representatives.

Defining Problem

The chief problem facing these sets of actors varies as well. For religious and secular elites like bishops and academic scientists, the primary challenges are winning contests of truth claims or expanding the boundaries of their institutions so that their values, priorities, and understandings orient the wider society. For ordinary people, it is "making a life" (Ammerman 2014) or cultivating habits and routines that infuse their everyday worlds with some overarching sense of purpose and significance. In contrast, for paid caregivers in the public sphere, the chief problem is to protect vulnerable strangers' essentially human qualities from rationalization by imbuing them with moral dignity and exceptional value and by making plausible those aspects of personhood, including the spiritual, that are denied or destabilized by rationalization.

Conception of Rationalization

These approaches also have different takes on Weber's notion of rationalization. One version of the secularization approach emphasizes the incompatibility of scientific and religious truth claims and invokes Weber's depiction of rationalization as a shell hard as steel (Baehr 2001). Here individuals are portrayed, like steel, as subject to a type of congealing process that changes them into radically altered and degraded forms of their prior selves. In this view, rationalization gets under people's skin and reconstitutes them as part human and part nonhuman. Like an armor-plated bug, they are reduced to the hardened outlook of the bourgeois philistine, incapable of aspiring to heaven or any nonutilitarian value. Another version of secularization theory imagines that rationalization won't change people in this fundamental way but will rob them of liberty. Instead of imagining rationalization as creating a "shell hard as steel," this version imagines it as an "iron cage" (Baehr 2001). This cage bars people from what Weber called "value rationality": outlooks that treat humanistic goals like compassion as inherently right and legitimate ends to pursue. This more popular version also emphasizes institutional differentiation: the iron cage of rationality, in this view, gets subdivided into more and more separate cells, each with its own distinct values, logics, and authority figures. In these different ways, both versions depict rationalization as ushering in a spiritually depleted epoch.

In stressing the relevance and transferability of spirituality to more mundane activities, the lived religion approach suggests that the essence of humanity remains intact within rationality's iron cage and that the cage can also be easily plied opened. Put differently, it agrees with Durkheim that the sacred and profane are alternative ways of understanding and interacting with the world but downplays his notion that there exists a sharp line between the two, suggesting that otherwise profane objects and activities might still be rendered sacred.

Unlike these two approaches, a caritas perspective emphasizes the indeterminate nature of rationalization. In other words, it's an open question whether public spaces will continue to allow for meanings that dignify humans. From a caritas perspective, the hard shell and iron cage of modernity may be porous. They may be subject to a kind of sintering process that infuses them with humanistic understandings just as metal can be infused with lubricants, creating more and less stable moral composites (see also Clegg and Lounsbury 2009). Such was the case, for example, with the nurses studied here who took spiritual practices developed outside public hospitals like being present with the sick and, depending on the circumstances and the degree to which they identified with their work role, integrated them with their scientific treatment of patients.

Characterization of Religion

Finally, these perspectives characterize religion differently. The secularization framework depicts religion as a set of beliefs about a supernatural reality and a distinct value sphere controlled by ecclesiastical authorities, both of which are endangered by naturalistic perspectives. Lived religion scholars suggest that religion consists of portable symbols and rituals such as sacred garments and prayer that enable individuals to affirm their faith by inducing deeply felt experiences of the holy in both their private and public lives. By comparison, a caritas perspective emphasizes the relational and person-affirming nature of religion (see also Latour 2005). In this perspective, the horizontal aspects of religion, which suggest that the holy can be found in "us," might be socially constructed, even in public contexts that threaten to depersonalize people, through interpersonal acts of care that dignify distressed strangers and reflect back to them sacred understandings of humanity.

In these ways, a care-centered perspective approaches the issue of religion's place in the public sphere differently. Secularization scholars are interested in whether religious authorities can impose their understandings on society. Lived religion researchers focus on whether people can experience the spiritual in ordinary everyday life. In contrast, the care-centered framework sketched here asks whether paid care providers can affirm the transcendent qualities of vulnerable strangers in rationalized, public settings that threaten to deny those qualities and thus dehumanize them. This question is vitally important because, while modernity has freed individuals to reject the advice of religious leaders and choose their own spiritual tribe, the fact remains that as a social species humans are inherently dependent on one another, and their willingness to expand or shrink circles of care depends on their capacity to imagine all persons as intrinsically valuable (see also Gilligan 1982; Held 2005).

POSSIBLE OBJECTIONS

Having suggested how our understanding of religion's public fate might build on this study's findings and its nascent framework, there are several objections that still need to be addressed. Critics might argue that because nurses' spiritual care can be rare and invisible, it is socially inconsequential. They would likely question the generalizability of this study's results to less religious countries of the West like the United Kingdom, France, and Denmark, where spirituality may be even less detectable and welcomed in the public sphere (Paley 2006). Critics might also point out that spirituality is not the only humanistic meaning, nor are nurses the only workers expected to provide a human touch. Indeed, compassion for others may be at stake and sorely tested by rationalization under many circumstances, such as the placement of refugees, asylum seekers, and undocumented migrants into government detention centers. And the same critics might argue that while incorporating an author's personal engagement with matters of suffering may help to provide context, those experiences are too subjective in nature and therefore have little scientific value.

In terms of the first objection, it is no doubt the case that affirming others' sacredness can be so infrequent and subtle as to barely register an effect on the social order. In the words of one resident chaplain, "How often do I feel I really connect with patients and make a difference? Maybe once a week, maybe once every two weeks, . . . I may go two weeks not feeling like I have connected at all." However, as other research demonstrates, many religious and spiritual movements of the past successfully changed nonsectarian institutions like businesses, schools, and governments by using unobtrusive, nonconfrontational tactics such as exposing them to contemplative culture or describing meditation using an organization's vernacular language (Kucinskas 2014). Out of the seedbed of these movements' spiritual practices new institutional structures often emerged. These practices were transformational because they were enacted within organizations' working, liminal spaces (e.g., lunchrooms, bathrooms, smoking lounges, stairwells) where actors seek refuge from turmoil, question their organization's taken-for-granted assumptions, and explore new perspectives (see also Shortt 2014).

In fact, small acts of caritas may be especially effective in otherwise morally sterile environments. The poet William Wordsworth spoke to this possibility when he wrote that "little, nameless, unremembered, acts of kindness and love" may form the "best portion of a good man's life." Just as the injuries of class can be hidden and lasting (Sennett and Cobb 1993), so, too, might the sanctity of strangers be invisibly repaired and sustained by inconspicuous, humanizing gestures. The word *sacrifice* comes from the Latin *sacer facer*—or "the making of the sacred." The "invisible" sacrifices that care workers make on behalf of suffering strangers may make them sacred, and in doing so may foster the development of societies that recognize the inherent dignity of all people (Schilling and Mellor 2013).[1]

As to whether this study's findings apply to less religious societies of the West, it is true that the United States and European countries occupy different points along the secularity spectrum. On virtually every measure, for example, religion in Britain is on the decline. Less than 10 percent of the population attends worship services or is a member of a church. Belief in a personal God also plummeted from 43 percent in the 1950s (Gill et al. 1998) to 26 percent by 2000 (Heald 2000). And yet, in the United Kingdom, as in the United States, interest in spirituality among nurses is quite high, judging by the rate of contributions to the "spirituality in nursing" literature

(Swinton and McSherry 2006). While it may be that nursing scholars are simply trying to expand the scope of their occupation's authority by capturing a newly recognized sphere of work, as some have claimed (Paley 2006), it may also be that British nurses are responding to patient needs that often go unacknowledged in a society lacking the types of cultural mechanisms examined here that make the spiritual plausible (Berger 1967, 45 and 192). If so, interest in spirituality among frontline care providers could ironically grow fastest in those parts of the world where traditional religious beliefs and participation are declining.

If the conceptual framework outlined here is to flourish, researchers need to examine the understandings, actors, and situations that bear on the ultimate worth of humans. In a society that often treats human beings as objects, humanistic meanings like spirituality support the sanctity of personhood. But rationalization doesn't just objectify human beings; it also dislocates them, isolates them, and disrupts their connection with history, undermining their sense of place, belonging, and continuity (Todres, Galvin, and Holloway 2009). The study of meanings that might counter these dangers may be especially relevant to settlement officers, rescue personnel, social workers, and teachers who directly care for refugees, victims of natural disasters, the homeless, and transient student populations.

These other humanistic meanings will become increasingly germane as countries deal with existential threats like climate change and war that test the bonds of unity and compassion for others. In recent dates, two conflicting forms of morality have become especially prevalent in the anglophone world: a *harm-based morality* focused on the virtues of caring, compassion, kindness, and protecting vulnerable others and an *in-group morality* focused on the threats posed by outsiders, refugees, foreigners, and immigrants (Wheeler, McGrath, and Haslam 2019). These conflicting moralities have been adopted by the political left and right, respectively. As the tension between these two outlooks intensifies, caritas will likely take center stage and the meanings attached to it will likely expand.

Readers will have to decide for themselves whether, in relaying personal experiences, I fell into the abyss of self-absorption, as scientific purists would have predicted, or skirted questions about the existence of the Divine, as religious fundamentalists might charge. A more relevant issue, though, may be what such disclosures say about social scientists' capacity to engage values of a personal nature. Having academics share their encounters with and responses to suffering helps, as some have argued (Kleinman 2020), to humanize social inquiry and integrate caregiving into academic discussions of social life. But such accounts could also be scientifically valuable in and of themselves. By systematically comparing them, we might learn more about how autobiography shapes the scientific process and, conversely, how the technical norms of science condition self-portraiture (Graham 2004). In some cases, writing about science and self might be quite compatible and can be seamlessly woven together. In other cases, such as in this book, accounts may be noticeably fragmented with several loose ends.

LOOKING FORWARD

While exploring the fate of caritas in public life, I stumbled upon some unexpected findings that seem worthy of further examination. As noted earlier, despite working in a setting where the phenomenon of suffering often brings spiritual concerns to the fore and being surrounded by coworkers who have a strong personal interest in spirituality, the topic rarely came up in conversations among nurses because they misperceived that such talk was unwanted. Equally striking, though, was how nurses responded when spirituality was discussed.

Many, like the head of the nursing division, neither questioned nor affirmed such talk but simply went along with it. "I happen to believe that whatever patients believe works for them, works for them. If they really believe that prayer is healing them, you know, I think the mind is a fascinating thing . . . and so if you really believe that prayer is going to heal you, then prayer can heal you." Similarly, another nurse said, "If they bring it [spirituality] up, I'll usually let them lead the conversation. I'll let them take it where they want to go with it. I don't offer any of critique. I would never tell anybody 'No, I don't believe that' or 'That's silly' or anything like that. That's part of their support system and I would never pull out the legs from somebody. So, if it's real to them, I treat it as if it were real to me." Others found spiritual talk amusing and were curious where it might lead. "There is only one nurse in our unit I know who talks about religion. He was raised Catholic and is a devout believer . . . I sometimes think his spirituality is kind of out there. Still, I try to listen to him. Sometimes you'll learn things if you just let them talk about what's on their mind." And still other nurses had their spiritual and scientific outlooks significantly altered and transformed when patients, especially those facing life and death circumstances, broached the topic, as we saw in the previous chapter.

These responses to spiritual talk, especially that of strangers, suggest the variety of ways that people talk about spirituality when it is brought out into the open. What's more, they offer clues about how such discourse might either weaken or restore a sense of the common good. Scholars have often dismissed language about self-fulfillment as vague and fuzzy, an expression of moral laziness, or a ruse created by a commodity culture that individualizes social problems and distracts our attention from politics. Yet, as some of these responses demonstrate, hearing the spiritual angst of strangers can sensitize listeners to what beyond themselves really matters (see also Frank 2002). Such a recognition may enable citizens to make the connection between personal problems and public issues, which is the foundation of politics (Mills 1959).

Another unanticipated finding is that large numbers of nurses associate spirituality with humor (see also Cain 2012). A full 89 percent of nurses disagreed or strongly disagreed with the statement "Spirituality has nothing to do with humor." In postsurvey interviews, some nurses explained that they considered certain spiritual practices to be absurd. One nurse commented,

> I guess whatever patients believe, I kind of have to also. I have to make accommodations because it is their support system. But it is not like I don't make jokes about these people when they're not around. I do. . . . There's people that have a lot of home remedies, such as shark cartilage. It's like a religion to them. I can't tell those people, "That shark cartilage, they are just taking your money." As much as I would like to, I have to be careful about that kind of stuff. I don't want to diminish their hope.

For others, spirituality was wrapped in dark humor. As an ICU nurse explained,

> Once a patient who was coding in our unit was visited by family members who kept telling her "It's okay to let go. It's okay to let go. Move toward the light. Move toward the light." Just as the patient's heart stopped, the computer monitor in the room shut off. The next few days that same computer did weird things, like go off and on in the middle of the night. Some of us said maybe her spirit got stuck in the computer and is rattling around

in there. To keep things upbeat, especially when we feel exhausted, we will sometimes say "Don't go toward the light! Don't go toward the light!" Or when a patient is dying, we will occasionally shine a flashlight on the wall to direct their spirit away from our equipment.

And according to yet others, laughter and spirituality were intertwined in moments of welcomed surprise. These nurses said their spirits were buoyed and mixed with laughter when patients' test results or medical procedures turned out better than expected. They also mentioned serendipitous experiences that, in their minds, hinted at wider horizons of meaning. Several nurses, for example, spoke of being moved and taken back by the high spirits of family members whose loved ones had passed or were about to. This response suggests that humor is not only part of a good life but also of spiritual value in itself. One nurse wrote,

> An older man was dying, he was a no code and placed in a private room. He was barely conscious and we were just doing comfort measures—turning, keeping him warm, etc. He had a huge family with 6 or 7 children and many grandchildren. When I first went into his room, I noticed all the family there were talking, laughing, and carrying on normal conversations around the patient. It dawned on me that they were providing the patient the best possible way to die, surrounding him with laughter, voices, and love. It's something I'll never forget—the feeling of inner peace that came over me.

It's not totally surprising that spirituality can be a source of humor in an academic medical center. After all, humor, by definition, usually involves a juxtaposition of dissimilar things. Weber did not talk about humor, and, in fact, he's often described as a touchy, gloomy character. But he wrote extensively about how human affliction heightens the tension between religion and science. Weber thought that as long as suffering remains an inevitable part of the human experience, people will be on the lookout for satisfying explanations of adversities, inequalities, and hardship. When they don't find those explanations in religion, they'll turn to scientific explanations—and vice versa. He thought that rationalization emerged, for example, because religions struggled to reconcile the problem of evil with belief in an omnipotent and benevolent God. This struggle led people to create secular spaces in the divine order where human affairs could be managed more rationally.

The explanations developed within these spaces eventually became dominant, suggesting that suffering could be solved through the power of reason.

But as time went on, rationalistic accounts struggled to reconcile their image of human progress with problems directly caused by human decisions, including the growing scale of warfare and environmental destruction. Now, their credibility, too, is being questioned. One result is a growing demand for sacred spaces within secular organizations, like the one studied here. It's not yet clear whether such spaces can be established and sustained. If they can, or if people end up toggling back and forth between religion and science, as I have, they'll be more exposed to the incongruities between sacred and rationalistic meanings and practices. Whether these incongruities lead them to dismiss spirituality as ludicrous or embrace it with a healing, postdoom laugh is a topic ripe for investigation.

FINAL THOUGHTS

As Weber suggested, the ongoing rationalization of modern society, with its focus on gaining ever more control over nature and people, threatens to trample the transcendent qualities of humanity standing in its path. In recent years, this danger has been amplified by the emergence of totalitarian movements like Christian nationalism that seek to reclaim the transcendent to reinforce religious and racial identities, foster a sense of victimhood, and justify attacks on democracy. Exacerbating this situation further is the growing influence of neoliberalism that valorizes individual autonomy and self-interest. While these developments have perhaps not caused people to care less than in the past, they dismiss the reality that human society is increasingly interdependent and erode the moral incentive to extend benevolence to strangers.

How long these violent and dehumanizing threats will last is unclear. What is clear is that it was only until the Axial Age, when moral universalism first appeared and the sanctity of all persons was recognized, that similar threats were reversed. This fact, coupled with the realization that society has not since developed an alternative basis for uniting humanity, suggests that the plight of vulnerable people will hinge on supporting the types of actors and developing the sorts of cultural supports examined here. They will ultimately determine whether the Axial principle of caritas becomes a social reality.

NOTES

1. RELIGION AND CARE OF THE STRANGER

1. At the time of the survey, University Hospital employed 597 full-time and part-time nurses.
2. This period has attracted considerable attention from a wide range of academic disciplines, including sociology (Bellah 2011; Bellah and Joas 2012), anthropology (Atran 2016), psychology (Boyer and Baumard 2016), philosophy (Habermas 2010), and history (Turchin 2015).
3. This relational understanding of spirituality also differs from what William James (1961) calls personal religion, mystical experiences that can occur regardless of organized religion or one's surrounding culture.
4. Transcendence here refers not to a place or some imaginable entity but to a nonspatial, nontemporal realm of meaning that is not directly accessible to human understanding but nonetheless imbues each individual with infinite value. This intimation of transcendence is compatible with every religious faith and philosophical or wisdom tradition that acknowledges an imperishable dimension of meaning. It is also compatible with agnostic sentiments and perspectives that recognize the ultimate mystery of human origins and purposes.
5. For a discussion of other regions in which this ethic might have emerged, see Mullins et al. (2018). As this study suggests, there are also debates among scholars about the causes and temporal boundaries of the Axial Age.
6. Even some atheists who reject the idea of an immortal soul grudgingly concede that the term *spirituality* captures a vital aspect of being human (Harris 2014; Sagan 1995). For related arguments on how secular society must frequently draw on religious language to specify values, see Steven Smith's *The Disenchantment of Secular Discourse* (2010).

7. As is the case with the concept of human rights (Łuków 2018), spirituality's underlying values are intentionally rendered vague, emphasizing instead the fragility of human existence and every person's participation in a transcendent reality.
8. According to one study (Mason et al., 2018), nurses have been used only 2 to 4 percent of the time as sources of quotations in articles about health care over the past two decades.
9. From their perspective, spirituality is at worst a type of pathology and at best a mild awe one might experience while gazing at a sunset.
10. I refer to this ethic as caritas here and elsewhere rather than employ the term Weber used more often, *brotherliness*, because of the latter's sexist overtones. The word *caritas* has its origin in the Hebrew word *ahabà* as it was used in the Torah to mean, broadly, a mature, loving, self-giving concern and care for other people, closely associated with the love of Yahweh for His people (Jackson 1999). When the Torah was translated from Hebrew into Greek during the third to first centuries BCE, *ahabà* was translated as *agapē*, spiritual love. As Christianity emerged and Latin became the dominant language, *agapē* was translated into Latin as *caritas*. In its origin, then, *agapē* or *caritas* is a Judeo-Christian concept. At the same time, *agapē* resonated with some nonreligious virtues, including empathy and compassion.
11. See also writings by Levinas (1995) on the face of the other.
12. See related writings by Niebuhr (2012) on caritas as the invaluable but "impossible possibility of love."
13. Slightly more than 50 percent (N = 299) of the 597 nurses in the hospital completed the survey; 36 of the remaining nurses were randomly selected for further follow-up. Only 1 of these 36 nurses ultimately refused, yielding a highly representative sample of the nonrespondents. The answers of the latter group were compared to those of the original 299 respondents on 270 close-ended survey items. The two groups differed significantly on only 11 questions (according to a t-test), which is less than 5 percent or what is conventionally expected because of pure chance, indicating that the sample for respondents was representative of the hospitals' entire nursing staff.

    The survey consisted of four sets of questions and one open-ended question: (1) a set of 20 questions regarding basic demographic characteristics; (2) a set of 83 questions about the types of patients and technologies nurses regularly work with; (3) a set of 87 questions on the nature of spirituality and its compatibility with modern medicine, including 20 items recently developed by the Fetzer Institute (1999) in collaboration with the National Institutes of Health (NIH); (4) a set of 80 questions developed by the researcher that asked nurses about which spiritual therapies they had ever offered, what they believe are the benefits of spirituality for patients, and the circumstances under which they have ever suggested, offered, or provided spiritual services to patients; and (5) an open-ended question that asked nurses to describe an event at work that greatly influenced their understanding of spirituality.
14. As Bauman (1972, 185) also suggests, "In the professional life of a sociologist his most intimate, private biography is inextricably entangled with the biography of his discipline; one thing the sociologist cannot transcend in his quest for objectivity is his own, intimate and subjective encounter-with-the-world."

15. The conflict between these two tasks will grow as neoliberalism erodes moral claims located outside capitalist rationality and devolves responsibility for sacralizing suffering individuals to overburdened and shrinking public agencies (see Bourdieu et al. 2010).

2. THE HISTORY OF CARITAS IN HEALTH CARE

1. In this section and the two that follow, I draw extensively on Ferngren's (2012) work on the historical relationship between medicine and religion.
2. The association of science with Greek culture is often overstated and ignores the influence of the Islamic world (see Majeed 2005).
3. See Agusti (2018).
4. For a review of research on spirituality in medicine, see Balboni and Peteet (2017).
5. When staff address the spiritual or religious concerns of internal medicine patients, patients are more likely to rate their care at the highest level on multiple measures of patient satisfaction (Williams et al. 2011). Alternately, patients whose spiritual needs are neglected give lower ratings of both quality of care and satisfaction with care (Astrow et al. 2007)

3. CRAFT VERSIONS OF RELIGIOUS AUTHORITY

1. See Norwood (2006).
2. Also, whereas from 1981 to 2007 there was an uptick in the number of individuals throughout the world who said God was important in their lives, since that period there has been a sharp decline in religiosity, especially in high-income countries (Inglehart 2020).

4. SECOND-GUESSING TALK ABOUT SPIRITUALITY

1. When studying absolute types of pluralistic ignorance, one sometimes confronts the problem of labeling the majority correctly. For example, if A says that "most persons hold belief Z" and only 49 percent do, A is in the WRONG category, while if 51 percent do, A is in the RIGHT category. There is no easy fix to this problem, but readers need to keep it in mind when interpreting distributions.

5. PATHWAYS TO SPIRITUAL MEANING AND EMOTIONAL DEAD ENDS

1. For a more in-depth discussion of this point, see Boltanski and Chiapello (2005).
2. For a related discussion of the quasi-religious aspects of organizational life, see Demerath (1999). Also, for a sampling of research on workplace spirituality by managerial scholars and more popular treatments of the subject, see Giacalone and

Jurkiewicz (2003), Mitroff and Denton (1999), Bolman and Deal (2011), and Alman, Neal, and Mayhofer (2022).

3. To be sure, not all students of emotional labor subscribe to an either/or understanding of emotional experiences (see Erickson 2007). Nor have all students skirted the issue of meaning (Kunda 1992).

4. Whether nurses' relationships with patients can be characterized as horizontal may depend on the relative power that patients are given to evaluate nurses. For the purposes of our discussion, though, this chapter treats these relationships as basically horizontal in nature.

5. On the difference between analytical propositions that are falsifiable and synthetic ones that are largely unfalsifiable, see Popper (1959).

6. In contrast, only 18.7 percent agreed and 5 percent strongly agreed with the statement that there is something "religious" about their care. And whereas there is a statistically nonsignificant correlation between the latter measure and our ($r = 0.093$), there is a statistically significant correlation between calling and our key dependent variable, "There is something spiritual about the care I provide" ($r = 0.269$).

7. See table A.5.3.

8. The reader may also notice that a factor can appear in more than one configuration. This suggests that the influence of a factor is most meaningfully understood as being contingent on the copresence of others. The reader may note that neither the presence nor the absence of trustworthy supervisors appears in any of the five configurations. This result indicates that the influence of this factor is already covered by another attribute in the solution. The fact that many supervisors are themselves nurses may also suggest that, in the minds of nurses, the counsel of a supervisor is not much different from the counsel received from peers.

9. These configurations' fuzzy-set scores are used to determine whether their membership in our solution terms has an effect above the main effects and controls (the latter two sets of variables are also fuzzified).

10. See table A.5.4.

11. See table A.5.5.

12. Table A.5.6 reports various percentiles of each configuration. These statistics suggest that while some configurations occur less often than others (e.g., configuration 5 is rarer than configuration 1), when configurations do occur, they matter a great deal.

13. As suggested earlier, that the hospital is affiliated with a public university and therefore is not entirely private may explain the small percentage of nurses who report feelings of inauthenticity.

14. See table A.5.7, which reports how consistently each configuration is associated with emotional inauthenticity. To be more exact, it determines how consistently each configuration is a subset of a fuzzified measure of emotional authenticity. We see that configurations 4 and 5 achieve what is considered a minimal level of consistency ($Y > 0.75$; Ragin 1987).

15. The analytical approach used here also shows how fsQCA provides the methodological legs that the negotiated order perspective needs to run on. If the approach proposed here is to prove useful, additional work is needed on other meanings than the ones examined here.

6. STYLES OF SPIRITUAL CARE

1. It could be that some nurses have fewer opportunities because they are overwhelmed by the number of patients they must care for, but, as noted earlier, in this particular hospital the nurse-to-patient ratio is capped at 1:4.
2. There is an ongoing debate within nursing about how spiritual care is be defined (McSherry and Draper 1998). In examining spiritual care, this chapter is not suggesting that it is equivalent to caring for what Goffman calls the sacred self, that it represents the full domain of patient-centered care, or even that it is the most important facet of it. Nor is it making any claims about whether nurses' spiritual care is right or wrong. Rather, it examines spiritual care to draw attention to the cultural dimensions of patient-centered care.
3. See also Durkheim (1912), who suggests that clans were the original sources of spiritual understandings.
4. See also Wuthnow's (1999) thesis that in today's secularized society, spiritual practices that can be applied in a variety of settings deepen individuals' relationship to the sacred in religious and nonreligious contexts.
5. Work orientations like calling, career, and job are not what identity theorists would categorize as role identities per se, but rather meld a role identity (e.g., nurse) with aspects of one's "person identities" or meanings that are "based on culturally recognized qualities, traits, and expectations" (Burke 2004, 9). As such, they suggest the prominence of the role identity within the self-concept.
6. In the case of nursing, a deeply caring self is also embedded in the culturally grounded conception of what it means to be a nurse.
7. In other models not reported here, career was used as the reference group. The results were the same for calling, with the one exception that it does not have a significant effect on religious circumstances.
8. In other models not reported here, career was used as the reference group, and it was discovered that calling still had significant effects on three outcomes.

7. BRIDGING SCIENCE AND SPIRITUALITY
THROUGH STORYTELLING

1. To get a better sense of how nurses understand spirituality and how it is operationalized here, refer to the section in the appendix to chapter 7 titled "Dependent Variables." The same techniques (Ragin 2000) used in earlier chapters are deployed here to determine the different combinations of rhetorical devices used by bedside nurses to portray spirituality favorably.
2. While studies of lived religion have offered several qualitative and quantitative techniques for examining spiritual experiences, they have struggled to incorporate these approaches into the same research design. In particular, they have lacked a method that can identify which combinations of rhetorical devices are necessary or sufficient for storytellers to cast their experiences in a largely positive, spiritual light.
3. As table A.7.2 indicates, initial results suggested that there are seven ways that nurses can render their work experiences in a positive, spiritual light. However, a comparison of cases that do and do not possess a particular rendering revealed that the sixth

and seventh renderings do not produce significantly higher scores on the dependent variable (see column titled "t-test").

4. Additional work is needed on how the experiences of other health care workers compare with those of nurses and how both groups critically evaluate experts' definitions of suffering.

8. RESTORING THE SANCTITY ONCE
BESTOWED ON HUMANITY

1. Simmel (2011) discusses how the diminution of sacrifice in the modern era as an irrational act has prompted a yearning for transcendence.

REFERENCES

Abbott, Andrew. 1988. *The System of Professions: An Essay on the Division of Expert Labor*. Chicago: University of Chicago Press.

Accad, Michael. 2016. "How Western Medicine Lost Its Soul." *Linacre Quarterly* 83, no. 2: 144–146. http://www.tandfonline.com/doi/abs/10.1080/00243639.2016.1169389.

Addams, Jane, and Ruth W. Messinger. 1999. *Twenty Years at Hull-House*. New York: Signet Classics.

Agusti, Alvar. 2018. "The Disease Model: Implications for Clinical Practice." *European Respiratory Journal* 51, no. 4: 1800188.

Alexander, J. 1990. "Differentiation Theory: Problems and Prospects." In *Differentiation Theory and Social Change: Comparative and Historical Perspectives*, ed. J. Alexander and P. Colomy, 1–15. New York: Columbia University Press.

Alexander, J. C., and P. Smith. 1993. "The Discourse of American Civil Society: A New Proposal for Cultural Studies." *Theory and Society* 22, no. 2: 151–207.

Allport, Gordon. 1924. *Social Psychology*. Boston: Houghton Mifflin.

Alman, Yochanan, Judi Neal, and Wolfgang Mayhofer. 2022. *Workplace Spirituality: Making a Difference (Management, Spirituality and Religion)*. Berlin: De Gruyter.

Ammerman, Nancy. 1997. "Golden Rule Christianity: Lived Religion in the American Mainstream" In *Lived Religion in America*, ed. David Hall, 196–216. Princeton, NJ: Princeton University Press.

Ammerman, Nancy T. 2006. *Everyday Religion: Observing Modern Religious Lives*. New York: Oxford University Press.

Ammerman, Nancy. 2013. *Sacred Stories, Spiritual Tribes: Finding Religion in Everyday Life*. New York: Oxford University Press.

Ammerman, Nancy. 2014. "Finding Religion in Everyday Life." *Sociology of Religion* 75, no. 2: 189–207.

Ammerman, Nancy. 2020. "Rethinking Religion: Toward a Practice Approach." *American Journal of Sociology* 126, no. 1: 6–51.

Appelbaum, Eileen, and Rosemary Batt. 1994. *The New American Workplace*. Ithaca, NY: ILR Press.

Armstrong, Karen. 2006. *The Great Transformation: The Beginning of our Religious Traditions*. New York: Anchor.

Armstrong, Karen. 2010. *Twelve Steps to a Compassionate Life*. New York: Anchor.

Asad, T. 2003. *Formations of the Secular: Christianity, Islam, Modernity*. Stanford, CA: Stanford University Press.

Ashforth, B., and D. Vaidyanath. 2002. "Work Organizations as Secular Religions." *Journal of Management Inquiry* 11, no. 4: 359–370.

Astrow, Alan, Ann Wexler, Kenneth Texeira, M. Kai He, and Danil Sulmasy. 2007. "Is Failure to Meet Spiritual Needs Associated with Cancer Patients' Perceptions of Quality of Care and Their Satisfaction with Care?" *Journal of Clinical Oncology* 25, no. 36: 5753–5757.

Atran, Scott. 2016. "Moralizing Religions: Prosocial or a Privilege of Wealth?" *Behavioral and Brain Sciences* 39: e2.

Baehr, Peter. 2001. "The 'Iron Cage' and the 'Shell as Hard as Steel': Parsons, Weber, and the Stahlhartes Gehause Metaphor in the Protestant Ethic and the Spirit of Capitalism." *History and Theory* 40, no. 2: 153–169.

Bailey, E. 1998. *Implicit Religion: An Introduction*. London: Middlesex University Press.

Balboni, M., and T. Balboni. 2018. *Hostility to Hospitality: Spirituality and Professional Socialization Within Medicine*. New York: Oxford University Press.

Balboni, Michael, and John Peteet, eds. 2017. *Spirituality and Religion Within the Culture of Medicine: From Evidence to Practice*. Oxford: Oxford University Press.

Barley, S. R., and G. Kunda. 2004. *Gurus, Hired Guns, and Warm Bodies*. Princeton, NJ: Princeton University Press.

Barnes, Michael H. 2009. *Stages of Thought: The Co-Evolution of Religious Thought and Science*. Oxford: Oxford University Press.

Barnum, Barbara Stevens. 2010. *Spirituality in Nursing: The Challenges of Complexity*. New York: Springer.

Baskin, K., and Dimitri M. Bondarenko. 2014. *The Axial Ages of World History: Lessons for the 21st Century*. Marblehead, MA: ISCE.

Bauman, Zygmunt. 1972. "Culture, Values and Science of Society." *University of Leeds Review* 15, no. 2: 185–203.

Bauman, Zygmunt. 2000. *Liquid Modernity*. Cambridge: Polity.

Becker, H., B. Geer, E. Hughes, and A. Strauss. 1976. *Boys in White: Student Culture in Medical School*. New York: Transaction.

Bell, E., and S. Taylor. 2003. "The Elevation of Work: Pastoral Power and the New Age Work Ethic." *Organization* 10, no. 2: 329–349.

Bellah, R. 1986. "Habits of the Heart: Implications for Religion." Presentation at St. Mark's Catholic, Isla Vista, California. February 21.

Bellah, R. 1999. "Max Weber and World-Denying Love: A Look at the Historical Sociology of Religion." *Journal of the American Academy of Religion* 67, no. 2: 277–304.

Bellah, Robert. 2011. *Religion in Human Evolution: From the Paleolithic to the Axial Age*. Cambridge, MA: Harvard University Press.

Bellah, Robert, and Hans Joas. 2012. *The Axial Age and Its Consequences*. Cambridge, MA: Harvard University Press.

Bellah, Robert, Richard Madsen, William Sullivan, Ann Swidler, and Steven Tipton. 1985. *Habits of the Heart: Individualism and Commitment in American Life*. Berkeley: University of California Press.

Bender, Courtney. 2003. *Heaven's Kitchen*. Chicago: University of Chicago Press.

Bender, C. 2010. *The New Metaphysicals: Spirituality and the American Religious Imagination*. Chicago: University of Chicago Press.

Bender, C., W. Cadge, P. Levitt, and D. Smilde, eds. 2013. *Religion on the Edge: De-Centering and Re-Centering Religion*. Oxford: Oxford University Press.

Bender, Courtney, and Ann Taves. 2012. *What Matters? Ethnographies of Value in a Not So Secular Age*. New York: Columbia University Press.

Berger, Peter. 1967. *The Sacred Canopy: Elements of a Sociological Theory of Religion*. New York: Anchor.

Berger, P., and T. Luckmann. 1966. *The Social Construction of Reality*. New York: Doubleday.

Besecke, Kelly. 2013. *You Can't Put God in a Box: Thoughtful Spirituality in a Rational Age*. Oxford: Oxford University Press.

Bolman, L., and T. Deal. 2011. *Leading with Soul: An Uncommon Journey of Spirit*. San Francisco, CA: Jossey-Bass.

Boltanski, Luc. 1999. *Distant Suffering: Morality, Media and Politics*. Cambridge: Cambridge University Press.

Boltanski, L., and E. Chiapello. 2005. *The New Spirit of Capitalism*. London: Verso.

Bone, Debora. 2002. "Dilemmas of Emotion Work in Nursing Under Market-Driven Health Care." *International Journal of Public Sector Management* 15, no. 2: 140–150.

Bourdieu, Pierre. 1977. *Outline of a Theory of Practice*. Cambridge: Cambridge University Press.

Bourdieu, Pierre. 2000. *The Weight of the World: Social Suffering in Contemporary Society*. Stanford, CA: Stanford University Press.

Bourdieu, P., G. Sapiro, P. Ferguson, R. Nice, and L. Wacquant. 2010. *Sociology Is a Martial Art: Political Writings by Pierre Bourdieu*. New York: New Press.

Boyer, Pascal, and Nicholas Baumard. 2016. "Projecting WEIRD Features on Ancient Religions." *Behavioral and Brain Sciences* 39: 23–24.

Bradshaw, A. 1997. "Teaching Spiritual Care to Nurses: An Alternative Approach." *International Journal of Palliative Nursing* 3, no. 1: 51–57.

Bradshaw, Ann. 2017. *The Nurse Apprentice, 1860–1977*. Abingdon, UK: Routledge.

Bradshaw, Ann. 1994. *Lighting the Lamp: Spiritual Dimension of Nursing Care*. Scutari.

Braverman, Harry. 1998. *Labor and Monopoly Capital: The Degradation of Work in the Twentieth Century*. New York: Monthly Press Review.

Brody, Howard. 2003. *Stories of Sickness*. New York: Oxford University Press.

Bromley, P., and W. Powell. 2012. "From Smoke and Mirrors to Walking the Talk: Decoupling in the Contemporary World." *Academy of Management Annals* 6, no. 1: 1–48.

Brooks, David. 2019. "What Makes Us All Radically Equal." *New York Times*, October 20, 2019.

Brown, Theresa. 2016. *The Shift: One Nurse, Twelve Hours, Four Patients' Lives*. Chapel Hill, NC: Algonquin.

Burawoy, Michael. 2005. "For Public Sociology." *American Sociological Review* 70, no. 1: 4–28.

Burke, P. 2004. "Identities and Social Structure: The 2003 Cooley-Mead Award Address." *Social Psychology Quarterly* 67, no. 1: 5–15.

Burke, P., and J. Stets. 2009. *Identity Theory*. New York: Oxford University Press.

Burkhart, Lisa and Nancy Hogan. 2008. "An Experiential Theory of Spiritual Care in Nursing Practice." *Qualitative Health Research* 18, no. 7: 928–938.

Burnum, B. 2010. *Spirituality in Nursing: The Challenges of Complexity*. 3rd ed. New York: Springer.

Cadge, Wendy. 2013. *Paging God: Religion in the Halls of Medicine*. Chicago: University of Chicago Press.

Cadge, W., E. H. Ecklund, and N. Short. 2009. "Religion and Spirituality: A Barrier and a Bridge in the Everyday Professional Work of Pediatric Physicians." *Social Problems* 56, no. 4: 702–721.

Cadge, W., and C. Hammonds. 2012. "Reconsidering Detached Concern: The Case of Intensive-Care Nurses." *Perspectives in Biology and Medicine* 55, no. 2: 266–282.

Cadge, Wendy, Peggy Levitt, and David Smilde. 2011. "De-Centering and Re-Centering: Rethinking Concepts and Methods in the Sociological Study of Religion." *Journal for the Scientific Study of Religion* 50, no. 3: 437–449.

Cadge, Wendy, and Michael Skaggs. 2019. "Humanizing Agents of Modern Capitalism? The Daily Work of Port Chaplains." *Sociology of Religion* 80, no. 1: 83–106.

Cain, Cindy. 2012. "Integrating Dark Humor and Compassion: Identities and Presentations of Self in the Front and Back Regions of Hospice." *Journal of Contemporary Ethnography* 41, no. 6: 668–694.

Camosy, Charles C. 2021. *Losing Our Dignity: How Secularized Medicine Is Undermining Fundamental Human Equality*. Hyde Park, NY: New City Press.

Cappon, Zanardi. 2020. "Spirituality: Can It Be a Key Tool for the Next Generation of Excellent Performers?" *Forbes*, November 3.

Casanova, Jose. 2012. *Public Religions in the Modern World*. Chicago: University of Chicago Press.

Catanzaro, A. M., and K. A. McMullen. 2001. "Increasing Nursing Students' Spiritual Sensitivity." *Nurse Education* 26, no. 5: 221–226.

Cauda, Edward. 1988. "Spirituality, Religious Diversity, and Social Work Practice." *Families in Society: The Journal of Contemporary Social Services* 69, no. 4: 238–247.

Chambliss, Daniel. 1996. *Beyond Caring: Hospitals, Nurses, and the Social Organization of Ethics*. Chicago: University of Chicago Press.

Charon, Rita. 2006. *Narrative Medicine: Honoring the Stories of Illness*. Oxford: Oxford University Press.

Chaves, Mark. 1993. "Intraorganizational Power and Internal Secularization in Protestant Denominations." *American Journal of Sociology* 99, no. 1: 1–48.

Chaves, Mark. 1994. "Secularization as Declining Religious Authority." *Social Forces* 72, no. 3: 749–774.

Chaves, Mark. 2010. "Rain Dances in the Dry Season: Overcoming the Religious Congruence Fallacy." *Journal for the Scientific Study of Religion* 49, no. 1: 1–14.

Chen, Carolyn. 2022. *Work Pray Code: When Work Becomes Religion in Silicon Valley*. Princeton, NJ: Princeton University Press.

Chopra, Deepak, and Leonard Mlodinow. 2012. *War of the Worldviews: Where Science and Spirituality Meet—and Do Not.* New York: Random House.

Christoff, Kalina. 2014. "Dehumanization in Organizational Settings: Some Scientific and Ethical Considerations." *Frontiers in Human Neuroscience* 8: 748.

Clark, C. C., J. R. Cross, D. M. Deane, and L. W. Lowry. 1991. "Spirituality: Integral to Quality Care." *Holistic Nursing Practice* 5, no. 3: 67–76.

Clegg, Stewart, and Michael Lounsbury. 2009. "Weber: Sintering the Iron Cage: Translation, Domination, and Rationality." In *The Oxford Handbook of Sociology and Organization Studies*, ed. Paul Adler, 118–145. Oxford: Oxford University Press.

Cobb, Mark, Christina Puchalski, and Bruce Rumbold, eds. 2012. *Oxford Textbook of Spirituality in Healthcare.* Oxford: Oxford University Press.

Cole, Teju. 2012. "The White-Savior Industrial Complex." *The Atlantic*, March 21.

Collins, Randall. 2004. *Interaction Ritual Chains.* Princeton, NJ: Princeton University Press.

Conlin, Michelle. 1999. "Religion in the Workplace: The Growing Presence of Spirituality in Corporate America." *Bloomberg*, November 1: 3–10.

Creed, W. E. D., Scully, M. A., and Austin, J. R. 2002. "Clothes Make the Person? The Tailoring of Legitimate Accounts and the Social Construction of Identity." *Organization Science* 13, no. 5: 475–496.

da Silva Borges, Muema, and Daniella Soares dos Santos. 2013. "The Field of Care: Quantum and Transpersonal Approach of Nursing Care." *Ciência Cuidado e Saúde* 12, no. 3: 606–611.

Dawkins, Richard. 2011. *The God Delusion.* Boston: Mariner.

de la Torre, Renée, and Cristina Gutiérrez Zúñiga. 2013. "Chicano Spirituality in the Construction of an Imagined Nation: Aztlán." *Social Compass* 60, no. 2: 218–235.

Demerath, N. J., III. 2000. "The Varieties of Sacred Experience: Finding the Sacred in a Secular Grove." *Journal for the Scientific Study of Religion* 39, no. 1: 1–11.

Dennett, Daniel. 2006. *Breaking the Spell: Religion as a Natural Phenomenon.* New York: Penguin.

Department of Health. 2003. *NHS Chaplaincy: Meeting the Religious and Spiritual Needs of Patients and Staff.* London: Department of Health.

Diers, Donna. 2004. *Speaking of Nursing: Narratives of Practice, Policy and the Profession.* Burlington, MA: Jones and Bartlett.

DiMaggio, Paul, and Walter Powell. 1983. "The Iron Cage Revisited: Isomorphism and Collective Rationality in Organizational Fields." *American Sociological Review* 48, no. 2: 147–160.

Dobbelaere, K. 1981. "Trend Report: Secularization: A Multi-Dimensional Concept." *Current Sociology* 29, no. 2: 3–153.

Dobbelaere, K. 1988. "Secularization, Pillarization, Religious Involvement, and Religious Change in the Low Countries." In *World Catholicism in Transition*, ed. T. M. Gannon, 80–115. London: Macmillan.

Drucker, P. 1995. *Managing in a Time of Great Change.* New York: Truman Talley.

Durkheim, Emile. 1951. *Suicide.* New York: Free Press.

du Toit, C. W. 2006. "Secular Spirituality Versus Secular Dualism: Towards Postsecular Holism as Model for a Natural Theology." *Theological Studies* 62, no. 4: 1251–1268.

Durkheim, Emile. 1912. *The Elementary Forms of Religious Life.* Cambridge, MA: Oxford University Press.

Durkheim, E. (1893) 1997. *The Division of Labor in Society*. New York: Free Press.

Eliasoph, Nina. 1998. *Avoiding Politics: How Americans Produce Apathy in Everyday Life*. Cambridge: Cambridge University Press.

Eliasoph, Nina, and Paul Lichterman. 2003. "Culture in Interaction." *American Journal of Sociology* 108, no. 4: 735–794.

Emerson, M., and D. Hartman. 2006. "The Rise of Religious Fundamentalism." *Annual Review of Sociology* 32, no. 1: 127–144.

England, P. 2005. "Emerging Theories of Care Work." *Annual Review of Sociology* 31, no. 1: 381–399.

Englehart, Katie. 2021. "'We Are Going to Keep You Safe, Even If It Kills Your Spirit.'" *New York Times*, February 19, 2021.

Epstein, R., and R. Street. 2011. "The Values and Value of Patient-Centered Care." *Annals of Family Medicine* 9, no. 2: 100–102.

Erickson, R. 1995. "The Importance of Authenticity for Self and Society." *Symbolic Interactionism* 18, no. 2: 121–144.

Erickson, R. 2007. "The Context of Care: Reconsidering Culture, Structure, and the Performance of Emotional Labor Among Registered Nurses." In *Social Structure and Emotion*, ed. Dawn T. Robinson and Jody Clay-Warner, 161–175. San Diego, CA: Elsevier.

Erickson, R., and W. Grove. 2008. "Emotional Labor and Health Care." *Sociology Compass* 2, no. 2: 704–733.

Erickson, R., and C. Ritter. 2001. "Emotional Labor, Burnout, and Inauthenticity: Does Gender Matter?" *Social Psychology Quarterly* 64, no. 2: 146–163.

Erickson, R., and A. Wharton. 1997. "Inauthenticity and Depression: Assessing the Consequences of Interactive Service Work." *Work and Occupations* 24, no. 2: 188–213.

Evans, John H. 2016. *What Is a Human? What the Answers Mean for Human Rights*. New York: Oxford University Press.

Evans, J. H., and M. S. Evans. 2008. "Religion and Science: Beyond the Epistemological Conflict Narrative." *Annual Review of Sociology* 34, no. 1: 87–105.

Fairman, Julie, and Patricia D'Antonio. 2008. "Reimagining Nursing's Place in the History of Clinical Practice." *Journal of the History of Medicine and Allied Sciences* 63, no. 4: 435–446.

Felder, M. M., H. H. van de Bovenkamp, M. M. Maaijen, and A. A. de Bont. 2018. "Together Alone: Organizing Integrated, Patient-Centered Primary Care in the Layered Institutional Context of Dutch Healthcare Governance." *Journal of Professions and Organization* 5, no. 2: 88–105.

Ferngren, Gary. 2012. "Medicine and Religion: A Historical Perspective." In *Oxford Textbook of Spirituality in Healthcare*, ed. Mark Cobb, Christina Puchalski, and Bruce Rumbold, 3–10. Oxford: Oxford University Press.

Fetzer Institute/National Institute of Aging. 1999. *Multidimensional Measurement of Religiousness/Spirituality for Use in Health Research: A Report of the Fetzer Institute /National Institute of Aging Working Group*. Kalamazoo, MI: Fetzer Institute.

Fetzer Institute. 2020. *What Does Spirituality Mean to Us?* https://fetzer.org/resources /what-does-spirituality-mean-us.

Fine, Gary. 1984. "Negotiated Orders and Organizational Cultures." *Annual Review of Sociology* 10: 239–262.

Fineman, S., ed. 1993. *Emotion in Organizations*. Newbury Park, CA: Sage.

Fiss, Peer C. 2007. "A Set-theoretic Approach to Organizational Configurations." *Academy of Management Review* 32: 1180-1198.

Fligstein, Neil. 1997. "Social Skill and the Theory of Fields." *Sociological Theory* 19, no. 2: 105-125.

Folbre, N. 2012. *For Love and Money: Care Provision in the United States*. New York: Russell Sage Foundation.

Frank, Arthur. 2002. "Why Study People's Stories? The Dialogical Ethics of Narrative Analysis." *International Journal of Qualitative Methods* 1, no. 1: 109-117.

Frank, Arthur. 2013. *The Wounded Storyteller: Body, Illness, and Ethics*. Chicago: University of Chicago Press.

Frank, Arthur. 2017. "An Illness of One's Own: Memoir as Art Form and Research as Witness." *Cogent Arts and Humanities* 4, no. 1: 1-7.

Frank, D., and J. Meyer. 2002. "The Profusion of Individual Roles and Identities in the Postwar Period." *Sociological Theory* 20, no. 1: 86-105.

Fromm, Erich. 1963. *The Dogma of Christ*. New York: Henry Holt.

Frye, Northrup. 1957. *Anatomy of Criticism*. Princeton, NJ: Princeton University Press.

Garcia, Katia, and Harold Koenig. 2013. "Re-Examining Definitions of Spirituality in Nursing Research." *Journal of Advanced Nursing* 69, no. 12: 2622-2634.

Giacalone, R., and C. Jurkiewicz, eds. 2003. *Handbook of Workplace Spirituality and Organizational Performance*. Armonk, NY: M. E. Sharpe.

Gill, A. 2001. "Religion and Comparative Politics." *Annual Review of Political Science* 4, no. 1: 117-138.

Gill, R., C. K. Hadaway, and P. L. Marler. 1998. "Is Religious Belief Declining in Britain?" *Journal for the Scientific Study of Religion* 37, no. 3: 507-516.

Gilligan, Carol. 1982. *In a Different Voice: Psychological Theory and Women's Development*. Cambridge, MA: Harvard University Press.

Gilligan, Carol. 2003. "Hearing the Difference: Theorizing Connection." *Anuario de Psicologia* 44, no. 2: 155-161.

Glenn, Evelyn Nakano. 2012. *Forced to Care: Coercion and Caregiving in America*. Cambridge, MA: Harvard University Press.

Goffman, Erving. 1956. "The Nature of Deference and Demeanor." *American Anthropologist* 58, no. 3: 475-499.

Goffman, Erving. 1961. *Asylums: Essays on the Social Situation of Mental Patients and Other Inmates*. New York: Anchor.

Gordon, Suzanne. 2006. *Nursing Against the Odds: How Health Care Cost Cutting, Media Stereotypes, and Medical Hubris Undermine Nurses and Patient Care*. Ithaca, NY: Cornell University Press.

Gordon, Suzanne. 2011. *When Chicken Soup Isn't Enough: Stories of Nurses Standing Up for Themselves, Their Patients, and Their Profession*. Ithaca, NY: ILR Press.

Gorski, Philip, and Samuel Nelson. 2013. "Conditions of Religious Belonging: Confessionalization, De-parochialization, and the Euro-American Divergence." *International Sociology* 29, no. 1: 1-19.

Gouldner, Alvin W. 1954. *Patterns of Industrial Bureaucracy*. Glencoe, IL: Free Press.

Graham, Leslie. 2004. "Scientific Autobiography: Some Characteristics of the Genre." *ASp* 43-44: 57-67.

Grant, Don, Alfonso Morales, and Jeffry Sallaz. 2009. "Pathways to Meaning: A New Approach to Studying Emotions at Work." *American Journal of Sociology* 115, no. 2: 327–364.

Greeley, Andrew. 1997. *Religion as Poetry.* New York: Transaction.

Greeley, Andrew, and Paul Sheatsley. 1971. "Attitudes Toward Racial Integration." *Scientific American* 225, no. 6: 13–19.

Greenwood, R., C. Oliver, R. Suddaby, and K. Sahlin-Andersson. 2007. *Sage Handbook of Organizational Institutionalism.* Newbury Park, CA: Sage.

Gutkind, Lee. 2014. *Many Sleepless Nights: The World of Organ Transplantation.* New York: Open Road Media.

Habermas, Jürgen. 2010. *An Awareness of What Is Missing: Faith and Reason in a Postsecular Age.* Cambridge: Polity.

Haidt, Jonathan. 2012. *The Righteous Mind: Why Good People Are Divided by Politics and Religion.* New York: Vintage.

Hallett, T. 2003. "Symbolic Power and Organizational Culture." *Sociological Theory* 21, no. 2: 128–149.

Hallett, Tim, and Marc Ventresca. 2006. "Inhabited Institutions: Social Interactions and Organizational Forms in Gouldner's Patterns of Industrial Bureaucracy." *Theory and Society* 35, no. 2: 213–236.

Handzo, George, Kevin Flannelly, and Brian Hughes. 2017. "Hospital Characteristics Affecting HealthCare Chaplaincy and the Provision of Chaplaincy Care in the United States: 2004 vs. 2016." *Journal of Pastoral Care and Counseling* 71, no. 3: 156–162.

Hanegraaff, W. J. 1999. "Defining Religion in Spite of History." In *The Pragmatics of Defining Religion: Contexts, Concepts and Contests,* ed. J. G. Platvoet and A. L. Molendijk, 337–378. Leiden: E. J. Brill.

Harrad, Rachel, Chiara Costentino, Robert Keasley, and Francesco Sulla. 2019. "Spiritual Care in Nursing: An Overview of the Measures Used to Assess Spiritual Care Provision and Related Factors Amongst Nurses." *Acta Biomedica* 90, no. 4: 44–55.

Harris, Sam. 2014. *Waking Up: Searching for Spirituality Without Religion.* New York: Simon and Schuster.

Haslam, N., and S. Loughnan. 2014. "Dehumanization and Infrahumanization." *Annual Review of Psychology* 65: 399–423.

Heald, G. 2000. *The Soul of Britain.* London: Opinion Research Business.

Heimer, Carol, and Lisa Staffen. 1998. *For the Sake of Children: Social Organization of Responsibility in the Hospital and the Home.* Chicago: University of Chicago Press.

Held, V. 2005. *The Ethics of Care: Personal, Political, and Global.* New York: Oxford University Press.

Henderson, V. 1973. *Basic Principles of Nursing Care.* Geneva: ICN.

Hennis, Wilhelm. 2000a. *Max Weber's Central Question,* trans. Keith Tribe. Newbury, UK: Threshold.

Hennis, Wilhelm. 2000b. *Max Weber's Science of Man: New Studies for a Biography of the Work,* trans. Keith Tribe. Newbury, UK: Threshold.

Herman, Carla. 2006. "Development and Testing of the Spiritual Needs Inventory for Patients near the End of Life." *Oncology Nursing Forum* 33, no. 4: 737–744.

Hochschild, Arlie. 1983. *The Managed Heart: The Commercialization of Human Feelings.* Berkeley: University of California Press.

Hochschild, Arlie. 2003. *The Commercialization of Intimate Life: Notes from Home and Work*. Berkeley: University of California Press.

Hondagneu-Sotelo, Pierrette. 2008. *God's Heart Has No Borders: How Religious Activists Are Working for Immigrant Rights*. Berkeley: University of California Press.

Hughes, E. C. 1958. *Men and Their Work*. Westport, CT: Greenwood.

ICN. 2000. *Code of Ethics for Nurses*. Geneva: International Council of Nurses.

Inglehart, Ronald. 2020. "Giving Up on God: The Global Decline of Religion." *Foreign Affairs*, September/October.

Jackson, T. P. 1999. *Love Disconsoled*. Cambridge: Cambridge University Press.

James, W. 1961. *The Varieties of Religious Experience*. New York: MacMillan.

Jaspers, Karl. 1953. *The Origin and Goal of History*, trans. Michael Bullock. London: Yale University Press.

Joas, Hans. 2013. *The Sacredness of the Person: A New Genealogy of Human Rights*. Washington, DC: Georgetown University Press.

Jones, Jeffrey M. 2021. "U.S. Church Membership Falls Below Majority for First Time." Gallup, March 29.

Kalberg, Stephen. 1990. "The Rationalization of Action in Max Weber's Sociology of Religion." *Sociological Theory* 8, no. 1: 58–84.

Kelley, R. 1985. *The Gold Collar Worker: Harnessing the Brain Power of the New Work Force*. Reading, MA: Addison-Wesley.

Kendrick, K. D., and S. Robinson. 2000. "Spirituality: Its Relevance and Purpose for Clinical Nursing in a New Millennium." *Journal of Clinical Nursing* 9, no. 5: 701–705.

Kim, C. S., D. A. Spahlinger, J. M. Kin, and J. E. Billi. 2006. "Lean Health Care: What Can Hospitals Learn from a World-Class Automaker?" *Journal of Hospital Medicine* 1, no. 3: 191–199.

Kleinman, A. 2007. *What Really Matters: Living a Moral Life Amidst Uncertainty and Danger*. Oxford: Oxford University Press.

Kleinman, A. 2012. "Caregiving as Moral Experience." *Lancet* 380, no. 9853: 1550–1551.

Kleinman, Arthur. 2020. *The Soul of Care: The Moral Education of a Husband and a Doctor*. New York: Penguin.

Kleinman, A., V. Das, and M. Lock, eds. 1997. *Social Suffering*. Berkeley: University of California Press.

Knapp S.J. 2016. "Weber and Levinas on Modernity and the Problem of Suffering: Reconstructing Social Theory as Ethically Framed Rather Than Epistemologically Framed." *Current Perspectives in Social Theory* 35: 145–170.

Korte, C. 1972. "Pluralistic Ignorance About Student Radicalism." *Sociometry* 35, no. 4: 576–587.

Kucinskas, Jaime. 2014. "The Unobtrusive Tactics of Religious Movements." *Sociology of Religion* 75, no. 4: 537–550.

Kucinskas, Jaime. 2018. *The Mindful Elite: Mobilizing from the Inside Out*. New York: Oxford University Press.

Kucinskas, J., B. Wright, D. Ray, and J. Ortberg. 2017. "States of Spiritual Awareness by Time, Activity, and Social Interaction." *Journal for the Scientific Study of Religion* 56, no. 2: 418–437.

Kunda, Gideon. 1992. *Engineering Culture*. Philadelphia: Temple University Press.

Kunda, G., and J. van Maanen. 1999. "Changing Scripts at Work: Managers and Professionals." *Annals of the American Academy of Political and Social Science* 561, no. 1: 64–80.

Latour, Bruno. 2005. " 'Thou Shall Not Freeze-Frame,' or, How Not to Misunderstand the Science and Religion Debate." In *Science, Religion, and the Human Experience*, ed. James D. Proctor, 27–48. Oxford: Oxford University Press.

Lawrence, Thomas, and Roy Suddaby. 2006. "Institutions and Institutional Work." In *Handbook of Organization Studies*, ed. S. R. Clegg, C. Hardy, T. B. Lawrence, and W. R. Nord, 215–254. 2nd ed. London: Sage.

Lawrence, Thomas, Roy Suddaby, and Bernard Leca. 2011. "Institutional Work: Refocusing Institutional Studies of Organization." *Journal of Management Inquiry* 20, no. 1: 52–58.

Lee, S. J. C. 2002. "In a Secular Spirit: Strategies of Clinical Pastoral Education." *Health Care Analysis* 10, no. 4: 339–356.

Leget, Carlo. 2022. "Humanist Approaches to Spiritual Care in Patient Counseling in the Netherlands." In *Suffering in Theology and Medical Ethics*, ed. Christof Mandry, 214–225. Leiden: E. J. Brill.

Leidner, R. 1993. *Fast Food, Fast Talk: Service Work and the Routinization of Everyday Life*. Berkeley: University of California Press.

Levett-Jones, T. L. 2007. "Facilitating Reflective Practice and Self-Assessment of Competence Through the Use of Narratives." *Nurse Education Practice* 7, no. 2: 112–199.

Levinas, Emmanuel. 1995. *Ethics and Infinity*. Livonia, MI: XanEdu.

Lindsay, Michael. 2007. *Faith in the Halls of Power: How Evangelicals Joined the American Elite*. New York: Oxford University Press.

Lively, K. J. 2006. "Emotions in the Workplace." In *Handbook of the Sociology of Emotions*, ed. Jan E. Stets and Jonathan H. Turner, 569–590. New York: Springer.

Lively, K. J., and D. R. Heise. 2004. "Sociological Realms of Emotional Experience." *American Journal of Sociology* 109, no. 5: 1109–1136.

Lo, M., and C. Stacey. 2008. "Beyond Cultural Competency: Bourdieu, Patients, and Clinical Encounters." *Sociology of Health and Illness* 30, no. 5: 741–755.

Lockhart, L., and F. Danis. 2010. *Domestic Violence: Intersectionality and Culturally Competent Practice*. New York: Columbia University Press

Lockner, Anne, and Chelsea Walcker. 2018. "The Healthcare Industry's Shift from Fee-for-Service to Value-Based Reimbursement." *Bloomberg Law*, September 26.

Longest, Kyle, and Stephen Vaisey. 2008. "Fuzzy: A Program for Performing Qualitative Comparative Analyses (QCA) in Stata." *Stata Journal* 8, no. 1: 79–104.

Lopez, Steven. 2006. "Emotional Labor and Organized Emotional Care: Conceptualizing Nursing Home Care Work." *Work and Occupations* 33, no. 2: 133–160.

Lucchetti, Giancarlo, Prieto Peres, Mario Fernando, and Rodolfo Furan Damiano, eds. 2019. *Spirituality, Religiousness and Health*. Cham, Switzerland: Springer.

Luckmann, T. 1967. *The Invisible Religion*. New York: MacMillan.

Łuków, Paweł. 2018. "A Difficult Legacy: Human Dignity as the Founding Value of Human Rights." *Human Rights Review* 19, no. 3: 313–329.

Majeed, Azeem. 2005. "How Islam Changed Medicine: Arab Physicians and Scholars Laid Basis for Medical Practice in Europe." *BMJ* 331, no. 7531: 1486–1487.

Mangione, Thomas M. 1995. *Mail Surveys: Improving Their Quality*. Thousand Oaks, CA: Sage.

Martin, J. 1992. *Cultures in Organizations*. Oxford: Oxford University Press.

Marx, Karl. 1867. *Capital: A Critique of Political Economy*. Hamburg: Otto Meissner.

Maslow, Abraham. 1998. *Maslow on Management*. Hoboken, NJ: Wiley.

Mason, Diana J., Barbara Glickstein, Laura Nixon, Kristi Westphaln, Sarah Han, and Kimberly Acquaviva. 2018. "The Woodhull Study Revisited: Nurses' Representation in Health News Media 20 Years Later." *Journal of Nursing Scholarship* 50, no. 6: 695–704.

Mathisen, J. 1992. "From Civil Religion to Folk Religion: The Case of American Sport." In *Human Kinetics*, ed. S. J. Hoffman. Champagne: University of Illinois Press.

Matthews, Dale, and Connie Clark. 1999. *The Faith Factor: Proof of the Healing Power of Prayer*. New York: Penguin.

Mayo, E. 1945. *The Social Problems of an Industrial Civilization*. Boston: Harvard University.

McClain, Colleen, Barry Rosenfeld, and William Breitbart. 2003. "Effect of Spiritual Well-Being on End-of-Life Despair in Terminally-Ill Cancer Patients." *Lancet* 361, no. 9369: 1602–1607.

McGlone, Em. 1990. "Healing the Spirit." *Holistic Nursing Practice* 4, no. 4: 77–84.

McGuire, Meredith. 1993. "Health and Spirituality as Contemporary Concerns." *Annals of the American Academy of Political and Social Science* 527, no. 1: 144–154.

McGuire, Meredith. 2008. *Lived Religion: Faith and Practice in Everyday Life*. New York: Oxford University Press.

McSherry, Wilfred. 1998. "Nurses' Perceptions of Spirituality and Spiritual Care." *Nursing Standard* 13, no. 4: 36–40.

McSherry, Wilfred and P. Draper. 1998. "The Debates Emerging from the Literature Surrounding the Concept of Spirituality as Applied to Nursing." *Journal of Advanced Nursing* 27, no. 4: 683–691.

McSherry, Wilfred, and Steve Jamieson. 2011. "An Online Survey of Nurses' Perceptions of Spirituality and Spiritual Care." *Journal of Clinical Nursing* 10, nos. 11–12: 1757–1767.

McSherry, Wilfred, and Linda Ross. 2002. "Dilemmas of Spiritual Assessment: Considerations for Nursing Practice." *Journal of Advancing Nursing* 38, no. 5: 479–488.

Merton, Robert. 1968. *Social Theory and Social Structure*. Glencoe, IL: Free Press.

Meyer, J., and B. Rowan. 1977. "Institutionalized Organizations: Formal Structures as a Myth and Ceremony." *American Journal of Sociology* 83, no. 2: 340–363.

Meyerson, D. 2003. *Tempered Radicals: How People Use Difference to Inspire Change at Work*. Cambridge, MA: Harvard Business School Press.

Miller, Dale, and C. McFarland. 1991. "When Social Comparison Goes Awry: The Case of Pluralistic Ignorance." In *Social Comparison: Contemporary Theory and Research*, ed. J. Suls and T. Wills, 287–313. Hillsdale, NJ: Erlbaum.

Mills, C. Wright. 1959. *Sociological Imagination*. Oxford: Oxford University Press.

Mitroff, I., and E. Denton. 1999. *A Spiritual Audit of Corporate America: A Hard Look at Spirituality, Religion, and Values in the Workplace*. New York: Jossey-Bass.

Mitzman, A. 1970. *The Iron Cage: An Historical Interpretation of Max Weber*. New Brunswick, NJ: Transaction.

Mohr, John. 1997. "Soldiers, Mothers, Tramps and Others: Discourse Roles in the 1907 New York City Charity Directory." *Poetics* 22, no. 4: 327–357.

Muirhead, R. 2004. *Just Work*. Cambridge, MA: Harvard University Press.

Mullins, Daniel Austin, Daniel Hoyer, Christina Collins, Thomas Currie, Kevin Feeney, Pieter François, Patrick Savage, Harvey Whitehouse, and Peter Turchin. 2018. "A Systematic Assessment of Axial Age Proposals Using Global Comparative Historical Evidence." *American Sociological Review* 83, no. 3: 596–626.

Mumby, D., and L. Putnam. 1992. "The Politics of Emotion: A Feminist Reading of Bounded Rationality." *Academy of Management Review* 17, no. 3: 465–486.

Nagai-Jacobsen, M. G., and M. A. Burkhardt. 1989. "Spirituality: Cornerstone of Holistic Nursing Practice." *Holistic Nursing Practice* 3, no. 3: 18–26.

Narayanasamy, A. 1999. "Learning Spiritual Dimensions of Care from a Historical Perspective." *Nurse Education Today* 19, no. 5: 386–395.

Narayanasamy, A., and J. Owens. 2001. "A Critical Incident Study of Nurses' Responses to the Spiritual Needs of Their Patients." *Journal of Advanced Nursing* 33, no. 4: 446–455.

Nash, L. 1999. *Believers in Business*. New York: Thomas Nelson.

Niebuhr, Reinhold. 2012. *An Interpretation of Christian Ethics*. Louisville, KY: Westminster John Knox Press.

Noelle-Neumann, Elizabeth. 1993. *The Spiral of Silence*. Chicago: University of Chicago Press.

Norris, Pippa, and Ronald Inglehart. 2004. *Sacred and Secular: Religion and Politics Worldwide*. New York: Cambridge University Press.

Norwood, Frances. 2006. "The Ambivalent Chaplain: Negotiating Structural and Ideological Difference on the Margins of Modern-Day Hospital Medicine." *Medical Anthropology* 25, no. 1: 1–29.

National Science Foundation. 2001. "Professional Ethical Rules for Nurses." ICN Ethical Rules. *NSF-The Series* nr. 2, Oslo.

O'Brien, Mary Elizabeth. 2010. *Spirituality in Nursing*, 4th ed. Sudbury, MA: Jones and Bartlett.

O'Gorman, Hubert. 1980. "False Consciousness of Kind: Pluralistic Ignorance Among the Aged." *Research on Aging* 2, no. 1: 105–128.

O'Gorman, Hubert. 1986. "The Discovery of Pluralistic Ignorance: An Ironic Lesson." *Journal of the History of the Behavioral Sciences* 22, no. 4: 333–347.

Oswick, Cliff. 2009. "Burgeoning Workplace Spirituality? A Textual Analysis of Momentum and Directions." *Journal of Management, Spirituality and Religion* 6, no. 1: 15–25.

Pache, Anne-Claire, and Filipe Santos. 2013. "Embedded in Hybrid Contexts: How Individuals in Organizations Respond to Competing Institutional Logics." *Research in the Sociology of Organizations* 39: 3–35.

Pagels, E. H. 1989. *Adam, Eve, and the Serpent: Sex and Politics in Early Christianity*. New York: Vintage.

Paley, John. 2006. "Spirituality and Secularization: Nursing and the Sociology of Religion." *Journal of Clinical Nursing* 17, no. 2: 175–186.

Pargament, Kenneth. 1997. *The Psychology of Religion and Coping: Theory, Research, and Practice*. New York: Guilford.

Pentaris, P. 2019. *Religious Literacy in Hospice Care: Challenges and Controversies*. London: Routledge.

Perrow, Charles. 1991. "A Society of Organizations." *Theory and Society* 20, no. 6: 725–762.

Peters, T., and R. Waterman. 1982. *In Search of Excellence: Lessons from America's Best-Run Companies*. New York: Harper and Row.

"PEW Religious Landscape Study." 2017. Washington, DC: PEW Research Center.

Popper, K. R. 1959. *The Logic of Scientific Discovery*. New York: Basic Books.

Powell, W., and P. DiMaggio, eds.1991. *The New Institutionalism in Organizational Analysis*. Chicago: University of Chicago Press.

Prentice, Deborah, and Dale Miller. 1993. "Pluralistic Ignorance and Alcohol Use on Campus: Some Consequences of Misperceiving the Social Norm." *Journal of Personality and Social Psychology* 64, no. 2: 243–256.

Raatikainen, R. 1997. "Nursing Care as a Calling." *Journal of Advanced Nursing* 25, no. 6: 1111–1115.

Ragin, Charles. 1987. *The Comparative Method*. Berkeley: University of California Press.

Ragin, Charles. 2000. *Fuzzy-Set Social Science*. Chicago: University of Chicago Press.

Ragin, Charles C., and John Sonnett. 2005. "Between Complexity and Parsimony: Limited Diversity, Counterfactual Cases, and Comparative Analysis." In *Vergleichen in der Politikwissenschaft*, ed. Sabine Kropp and Michael Minkenberg. Wiesbaden: VS Verlag für Sozialwissenschaften.

Rainie, Lee, Scott Keeter, and Andrew Perrin. 2019. "Trust and Distrust in America." Washington, DC: PEW Research Center.

Reed, Pamela. 1996. "Transcendence: Formulating Nursing Perspectives." *Nursing Science Quarterly* 9, no. 1: 2–4.

Reich, Adam. 2014. *Selling Our Souls: The Commodification of Hospital Care in the United States*. Princeton, NJ: Princeton University Press.

Reinert, Katia Garcia and Harold Koenig, 2013 "Re-Examining Definitions of Definitions of Spirituality in Nursing Research." *Journal of Advanced Nursing* 69, no. 12: 2622–34.

Reinhart, R. J. 2020. "Nurses Continue to Rate Highest in Honesty, Ethics." Gallup.

Ricouer, Paul. 1958. "Ye Are the Salt of the Earth." *Ecumenical Review* 10, no. 3: 264–276.

Riesebrodt, Martin. 2010. *The Promise of Salvation: A Theory of Religion*. Chicago: University of Chicago Press.

Robinson, Marilynne. 2012. *When I Was a Child I Read Books: Essays*. New York: Farrar, Straus and Giroux.

Roof, Wade Clark 1993. *A Generation of Seekers: The Spiritual Journey of the Baby Boom Generation*. San Francisco, CA: Harper and Row.

Roof, Wade Clark. 1999. *Spiritual Marketplace: Babyboomers and the Remaking of American Religion*. Princeton, NJ: Princeton University Press.

Rosenberg, Charles. 1987. *The Care of Strangers: The Rise of America's Hospital System*. New York: Basic Books.

Ross, L. 1994. "Spiritual Aspects of Nursing." *Journal of Advanced Nursing* 19, no. 30: 439–447.

Ross, L. 2006. "Spiritual Care in Nursing: An Overview of the Research to Date." *Journal of Clinical Nursing* 15, no. 7: 852–862.

Saad, Marcelo, Roberto de Medeiros, and Amanda Mosini. 2017. "Are We Ready for a True Biopsychosocial-Spiritual Model? The Many Meanings of 'Spiritual.'" *Medicines* (Basel) 4, no. 4: 79.

Sagan, Carl. 1995. *The Demon-Haunted World*. New York: Random House.

Scheper-Hughes, Nancy. 1992. *Death Without Weeping: The Violence of Everyday Life in Brazil*. Berkeley: University of California Press.

Schuman, Howard, Charlotte Steeh, and Lawrence Bobo. 1985. *Racial Attitudes in America*. Cambridge, MA: Harvard University Press.

Schwalbe, M. L. 1993. "Goffman Against Postmodernism: Emotion and the Reality of the Self." *Symbolic Interaction* 16, no. 4: 333–350.

Scott, W. R., M. Ruef, P. Mendel, and C. Coronna. 2000. *Institutional Change and Healthcare Organizations*. Chicago: University of Chicago Press.

Seidman, S. 1985. "Modernity and the Problem of Meaning: The Durkheimian Tradition." *Sociological Analysis* 46, no. 2: 109–130.

Sennett, Richard, and Jonathan Cobb. 1993. *The Hidden Injuries of Class*. New York: W. W. Norton.

Serpa, S., and C. M. Ferreira. 2019. The Concept of *Bureaucracy* by Max Weber. *International Journal of Social Science Studies* 7, no. 2: 12–18.

Seybolt, Taylor. 2008. *Humanitarian Military Intervention: The Conditions for Success and Failure*. Oxford: Oxford University Press.

Shallenberger, D. 1996. "Reclaiming the Spirit: The Journeys of Gay Men and Lesbian Women Toward Integration." *Qualitative Sociology* 19, no. 2: 195–215.

Shamir, Jacob, and Michal Shamir. 1997. "Pluralistic Ignorance Across Issues and over Time: Information Cues and Biases." *Public Opinion Quarterly* 61, no. 2: 227–260.

Sherman, R. 2014. "Caring or Catering: Emotions, Autonomy, and Subordination in Lifestyle Work." In *Caring on the Clock: The Complexities and Contradictions of Paid Care Work*, ed. M. Duffy, A. Armenia, and C. Stacey. New Brunswick, NJ: Rutgers University Press.

Shilling, Chris and Philip Mellor. 2013. "'Making Things Sacred': Re-Theorizing the Nature and Function of Sacrifice in Modernity." *Journal of Classical Sociology* 13, no. 3: 319–337.

Shortt, Harriet. 2014. "Liminality, Space and the Importance of 'Transitory Dwelling Places' at Work." *Human Relations* 68, no. 4: 633–658.

Showers, F. 2014. "Building a Professional Identity: Boundary Work and Meaning Making Among West African Immigrant Nurses." In *Caring on the Clock: The Complexities and Contradictions of Paid Care Work*, ed. M. Duffy, A. Armenia, and C. Stacey. New Brunswick, NJ: Rutgers University Press.

Simmel, Georg. 1950. *The Sociology of Georg Simmel*. Glencoe, IL: Free Press.

Simmel, Georg. 2011. *The View of Life*. Chicago: University of Chicago Press.

Slack, Paul. 2012. *Plague: A Very Short Introduction*. Oxford: Oxford University Press.

Smith, Steven. 2010. *The Disenchantment of Secular Discourse*. Cambridge, MA: Harvard University Press.

Snead, O. C. 2020. *What It Means to Be Human*. Cambridge: Cambridge University Press.

Snow, D., and R. Machalek. 1982. "On the Presumed Fragility of Unconventional Beliefs." *Journal for the Scientific Study of Religion* 21, no. 1: 15–26.

Solari, C. 2006. "Professionals and Saints: How Immigrant Careworkers Negotiate Gender Identities at Work." *Gender and Society* 20, no. 3: 301–331.

Solari-Twadell, P. Ann, and Deborah Ziebarth, eds. 2020. *Faith Community Nursing*. Cham, Switzerland: Springer.

Solomon, R. 2002. *Spirituality for the Skeptic: The Thoughtful Love of Life*. New York: Oxford University Press.

Stacey, C. 2011. *The Caring Self: The Work Experiences of Home Care Aides*. Ithaca, NY: Cornell/ILR Press.

Starr, P. 1982. *The Social Transformation of American Medicine*. New York: Basic Books.

"State of the Church 2020." 2020. Barna.

Stets, J., and M. Carter. 2012. "A Theory of the Self for the Sociology of Morality." *American Sociological Review* 77, no. 1: 120–140.

Stone, Deborah. 2000. "Caring by the Book." In *Care Work: Gender, Labor, and the Welfare State*, ed. Madonna Harrington Meyer, 89–111. New York: Routledge.

Stranahan, S. 2001. "Spiritual Perception, Attitudes About Spiritual Care, and Spiritual Care Practices Among Nurse Practitioners." *Western Journal of Nursing Research* 23, no. 1: 90–104.

Strauss, A., S. Fagerhaugh, B. Suczek, and C. Wiener. 1982. "Sentimental Work in the Technologized Hospital." *Sociology of Health and Illness* 4, no. 3: 254–278.

Strauss, A., L. Schatzman, D. Erlich, R. Bucher, and M. Sabshin. 1963. "The Hospital and Its Negotiated Order." In *The Hospital in Modern Society*, ed. E. Friedson, 147–169. New York: Free Press.

Stryker, Sheldon. 1980. *Symbolic Interactionism: A Social Structural Version*. Menlo Park, CA: Benjamin Cummings.

Sullivan, Winnifred Fallers. 2014. *A Ministry of Presence: Chaplaincy, Spiritual Care, and the Law*. Chicago: University of Chicago Press.

Sullivan, Winnifred Fallers, E. Hurd, S. Mahmood, and P. Danchin, eds. 2015. *Politics of Religious Freedom*. Chicago: University of Chicago Press.

Sulmasy, Daniel. 2007. *The Rebirth of the Clinic: An Introduction to Spirituality in Health Care*. Washington, DC: Georgetown University Press.

Swidler, Ann. 1986. "Culture in Action: Symbols and Strategies." *American Sociological Review* 51, no. 2: 273–286.

Swinton, John, and Wilfred McSherry. 2006. "Critical Reflections on the Current State of Spirituality-in-Nursing." *Journal of Clinical Nursing* 15, no. 7: 801–802.

Symonds, Michael. 2016. *Max Weber's Theory of Modernity: The Endless Pursuit of Meaning*. New York: Routledge.

Symonds, Michael, and Jason Pudsey. 2006. "The Forms of Brotherly Love in Max Weber's Sociology of Religion." *Sociological Theory* 24, no. 2: 133–149.

Tada, Mitsuhiro. 2018. "Language, Ethnicity, and the Nation-State: On Max Weber's Conception of 'Imagined Linguistic Community.'" *Theoretical Sociology* 47, no. 4: 437–466.

Tang, Yijie. 2016. "Repositioning Confucianism in a New 'Axial Age.'" In *Anthology of Philosophical and Cultural Issues*, 85–92. Singapore: Springer Singapore.

Taylor, C. 1989. *The Ethics of Authenticity*. Cambridge, MA: Harvard University Press.

Taylor, Charles. 2007. *A Secular Age*. Cambridge, MA: Harvard University Press.

Taylor, E. 2012. *Religion: A Clinical Guide for Nurses*. New York: Springer.

Taylor, E. J., M. Amenta, and M. Highfield. 1995. "Spiritual Care Practices of Oncology Nurses." *Oncology Nursing Forum* 22, no. 1: 31–39.

Taylor, E. J., M. F. Highland, and M. Amenta. 1999. "Predictors of Oncology and Hospice Nurses' Spiritual Care Perspectives and Practices." *Applied Nursing Research* 12, no. 1: 30–37.

Taylor, Elizabeth, and Iris Mamier. 2005. "Spiritual Care Nursing: What Cancer Patients and Family Caregivers Want." *Journal of Advanced Nursing* 49, no. 3: 260–267.

Taylor, Elizabeth Johnston, and Myrna Trippon. 2020. "What Chaplains Wish Nurses Knew: Findings from an Online Survey." *Holistic Nursing Care* 34, no. 5: 266–273.

Taylor, Phyllis, and Ginette Ferszt. 1990. "Spiritual Healing." *Holistic Nursing Practice* 4, no. 4: 32–38.

Taylor, Verta. 1989. "Social Movement Continuity: The Women's Movement in Abeyance." *American Sociological Review* 54, no. 5: 761–775.

Ten Dam, Eline, and Maikel Waardenburg. 2020. "Logic Fluidity: How Frontline Professionals Use Institutional Logics in Their Day-to-Day Work." *Journal of Professions and Organization* 7, no. 2: 188–204.

Tillich, Paul. 1945. "Vertical and Horizontal Thinking." *American Scholar* 15, no. 1: 102–105.

Todres, L., K. Galvin, and I. Holloway. 2009. "The Humanization of Health Care: A Value Framework for Qualitative Research." *International Journal of Qualitative Studies on Health and Well-Being* 4, no. 2: 68–77.

Tronto, Joan. 1993. *Moral Boundaries: A Political Argument for an Ethic of Care*. New York: Routledge.

Tronto, Joan. 2013. *Caring Democracy: Markets, Equality, and Justice*. New York: New York University Press.

Turchin, Peter. 2015. *Ultrasociety: How 10,000 Years of War Made Humans the Greatest Cooperators on Earth*. Chaplin, CT: Beresta Books.

Turner, Bryan. 2017. "Ritual, Belief and Habituation: Religion and Religions from the Axial Age to the Anthropocene." *European Journal of Social Theory* 20, no. 1: 132–145.

United Kingdom Central Council for Nursing, Midwifery and Health Visiting (UKCC). 2000. *Requirements for Pre-Registration Nursing Programmes*. London: UKCC.

VandeCreek, Larry. 2003. *Professional Chaplaincy and Clinical Pastoral Education Should Become More Scientific*. Milton Park, UK: Routledge.

Walter, T. 1997. "The Ideology and Organization of Spiritual Care: Three Approaches." *Palliative Medicine* 11, no. 1: 21–30.

Warner, R. Stephen. 1988. *New Wine in Old Wineskins*. Berkeley: University of California Press.

Watson, M. Jean. 1988. "New Dimensions of Human Caring Theory." *Nursing Science Quarterly* 1, no. 4: 175–181.

Watts, Galen, and Dick Houtman. 2022. "The Spiritual Turn and the Disenchantment of the World: Max Weber, Peter Berger and the Religion–Science Conflict." *Sociological Review* May: 1–19.

Weber, Max. 1949. *The Methodology of the Social Sciences*. Glencoe, IL: Free Press.

Weber, Max. (1946) 1958a. *From Max Weber: Essays in Sociology*, ed. and trans. H. H. Gerth and C. Wright Mills. New York: Oxford University Press.

Weber, Max. (1946) 1958b. "Politics as a Vocation." In Gerth and Mills, *From Max Weber: Essays in Sociology*.

Weber, Max. (1904) 1958c. *The Protestant Ethic and the Spirit of Capitalism*. New York: Charles Scribner.

Weber, Max. (1946) 1958d. "Religious Rejections of the World and Their Directions." In Gerth and Mills, *From Max Weber: Essays in Sociology*.

Weber, Max. (1946) 1958e. "Science as a Vocation." In Gerth and Mills, *From Max Weber: Essays in Sociology*.

Weber, Max. (1968) 1978. *Economy and Society: An Outline of Interpretive Sociology*. Berkeley: University of California Press.

Weber, Max. (1895) 1980. "The National State and Economic Policy (Freiburg Address)." *Economy and Society* 9, no. 4: 428–449.

Weiner, A., and J. Ronch, eds. 2003. *Culture Change in Long-Term Care*. Binghamton, NY: Haworth.

Wheeler, M. A., M. J. McGrath, and N. Haslam. 2019. "Twentieth Century Morality: The Rise and Fall of Moral Concepts from 1900 to 2007." *PLoS ONE*, 14, no. 2: e0212267.

Whyte, William H. 1956. *The Organization Man*. Garden City, NJ: Doubleday.

Wilcox, Melissa. 2009. *Queer Women and Religious Individualism*. Bloomington: Indiana University Press.

Wilkinson, Iain. 2013. "The Problem of Suffering as a Driving Force of Rationalization and Social Change." *British Journal of Sociology* 64, no. 1: 123–141.

Wilkinson, Iain, and Arthur Kleinman. 2016. *Passion for Society: How We Think About Suffering*. Berkeley: University of California Press.

Williams, Joshua, David Meltzer, Vineet Arora, Grace Chung, and Farr Curlin. 2011. "Attention to Inpatients' Religious and Spiritual Concerns: Predictors and Association with Patient Satisfaction." *Journal of General Internal Medicine* 26, no. 11: 1265–1271.

Wilson, Bryan. 1976. *Contemporary Transformations of Religion*. Oxford: Oxford University Press.

Woodward, K. 2002. "Calculating Compassion." *Indiana Law Journal* 77, no. 2: 223–245.

Wright, Andrew. 2000. *Spirituality and Education*. London: Routledge.

Wuthnow, Robert. 1992. *Rediscovering the Sacred: Perspectives on Religion in Contemporary Society*. Grand Rapids, MI: William B. Eerdmans.

Wuthnow, Robert. 1993. *Acts of Compassion: Caring for Others and Helping Ourselves*. Princeton, NJ: Princeton University Press.

Wuthnow, Robert. 1999. *After Heaven: Spirituality in America Since the 1950s*. Berkeley: University of California Press.

Wuthnow, Robert. 2011. "Taking Talk Seriously: Religious Discourse as Social Practice." *Journal for the Scientific Study of Religion* 50, no. 1: 1–21.

Wuthnow, Robert. 2012. *The God Problem: Expressing Faith and Being Reasonable*. Berkeley: University of California Press.

Yam, B. M. 2004. "From Vocation to Profession: The Quest for Professionalization of Nursing." *British Journal of Nursing* 13, no. 16: 978–982.

Yamane, D. 1997. "Secularization on Trial: In Defense of a Neosecularization Paradigm." *Journal for the Scientific Study of Religion* 36, no. 1: 109–122.

Zelizer, Viviana A. Rotman. 2017. *Morals and Markets: The Development of Life Insurance in the United States*. New York: Columbia University Press.

INDEX

Page numbers in *italics* indicate figures or tables.

Abbott, Andrew, 71, 78–79

absolute pluralistic ignorance, 97

academic medical centers: chaplains in, 29, 72–73; detotalizing philosophy of patient-centered care, 149; holistic care at, 5; medical research and education at, 47; Medicare and Medicaid for, 48; Medicare payment reductions to, 73; overburdened work environment of, 84; poverty and, 47–48; public funding of, 30, 48; as rationalized institution, 30

actions: caritas through, 7, 29, 31, 37, 206; Weber on caritas routine, 37; Weber on social, 146. *See also* spiritual care styles

actors: ethic of caritas, 206–207; humanity and sanctity restoration, 211–212

Addams, Jane, 27

Aeschylus, 45

affirmation, of care for strangers, 28

agape (spiritual love), 222n10

ahaba (spiritual love), 222n10

Allport, Floyd on, 98

almshouses, 34–35

alternative therapies, nursing and, 53

altruistic universalism, in Axial Age, 12

ancient religions: Ferngren on, 43–44; illness treatment by, 44; on retributive misfortune, 34, 44

anthropocentrism: Dawkins biological, 15; Evans on, 15; Singer philosophical, 15; theological Judeo-Christian, 15

Aquinas, Thomas, 49

Aristotle, 183

Armstrong, Karen, 45

authenticity, 120–121, 125, 133–134; emotionally authenticating spiritualism, 139

authority: Abbott on craft-based, 71, 78–79; caritas through, 7, 29, 31, 206; chaplains spiritual care, 48; distrust of, 76–77. *See also* religious authority

Axial Age (800–200 BCE), 13; altruistic universalism in, 12; care for strangers as religious value, 5; Christianity and, 45–46; figures associated with,

Axial Age (800–200 BCE) (*continued*)
23; humanity spiritual development,
11; Islam and, 45–46; Jaspers on,
22; Rabbinic Judaism and, 45–46;
religious movements in, 11; spiritual
dignity advocacy, 5, 11–12; suffering as
opportunity to provide care, 45
Axial ethic, 221n5; modern relevance of,
14–16

Balanced Budget Amendments (1997),
Medicare payments reductions to
academic medical centers, 73
Bellah, Robert, 23–24
Bender, Courtney, 9
biological anthropocentrism,
of Dawkins, 15
biomedicine, 48, 180; body-soul analogy
dismissal, 49; Descartes and, 49;
McClain, Rosenfeld, Breitbart
spirituality and, 49; pathology
focus, 49
biopsychosocial model of health,
49, 50, 167
body-soul analogy: Aquinas on, 49;
biomedicine dismissal of, 49; of Greek
medicine, 44, 45, 49
bound in relationships storytelling
theme, *191*, 192
Breitbart, William, 49
Brooks, David, 14–15
brotherliness, Weber on, 17, 222n10

Cadge, Wendy, 48
calling work orientation, 159, 161–162,
162–166, 169, 225n5, 225n7
capitalism, Marx on poverty and, 25
care: frontline staff responsibility for
human spirit, 14, 24; group and
worthiness of, 11; person-centered
approach to, 53–54; salvation religions
ethics for, 17
care-centered perspective, 214
career work orientation, 159, 161, *162–166*,
225n5, 225n7
care for strangers: affirmation of, 28;
Axial Age religious value of, 5;

professionalism and, 149–151; public
religion for, 6–7; as religious value,
5, 8, 13
caregivers: care for strangers, 6;
emotional well-being, 132; moral
dilemmas of, 25; professionalism
and, 150–151; as spiritual but not
religious, 24
caritas (love for all people), 6, *211*;
through actions, 7, 29, 31, 37, 206;
through authority, 7, 29, 31, 206;
durability in modern era, 38; through
emotions, 7, 29, 31, 206; history of
conflict between rationalization and,
11–12; hospital loose coupling of, 8;
as Judeo-Christian concept, 222n10;
through language, 7, 29, 31, 206;
meaning of, 9; through narrative, 7,
29, 31, 206; organizational expressions
of, 46–48; scholars on fate of, 22–24;
secularization perspective neglect of,
209–210; social significance of, 38;
spiritual dimension of, 9, 203, 222n10;
Weber on fate of, 22–24; Weber on
rationalization threat to, 7, 18–19, 209,
220; Weber on routine action of, 37.
See also historical development, of
caritas
caritas-centered perspective, 38, 213
centripetal and centrifugal framings
rhetorical device, 183, 184, *190*, *195*,
195–197
chaplain intern experience, 38, 39–40,
43; CPE and, 66, 68, 69–70,
90–92, 143–144; social justice and,
42; spiritual care styles and, 143–145;
spirituality discussion and, 90–93;
spiritual meaning pathways and,
118–120; storytelling and, 173–176;
on Weber world disenchantment,
41–42
chaplains: in academic medical centers,
29, 72–73; Cadge on certification
of, 48; cost-cutting of, 75–76; nurse
opinions on becoming surrogate,
81–84; Rogerian therapy approach, 69,
92, 119, 144; spiritual care authority

of, 48; University Hospital program termination, 71, 74, 85, 204

Christianity: Axial Age and, 45–46; bridging role, 207; care to sick of, 34. *See also* Judeo-Christian concept

Christoff, Kalina, 16

Clinical Pastoral Education (CPE), in hospitals, 48, 72, 73; chaplain intern experience and, 66, 68, 69–70, 90–92, 143–144; IRS seminar of, 92, 118–119; seminars for, 92

Code of Ethics, of ICN, 54

code of ethics, on nurse spiritual care, 54

cognitive frames, in negotiated orders, 130–131

compassion: faith traditions code of, 17; Greek medicine understanding of suffering and, 45

controversies, over modern care systems, 23

corporate-sponsored spiritual meanings: emotions at work, 122–124; Weber on rationalization meaningless effect, 124–127

countertrends, in secularization, 76–78

COVID-19 patients, frontline staff and, 14

CPE. *See* Clinical Pastoral Education

craft-based authority, 86; Abbott on, 71, 78–79

culture: of patient-centered models, 152; pluralistic ignorance and organization, 101; Weber on, 30–31

Dawkins, Richard, 15

dehumanization: Christoff on mechanical, 16; human suffering, 26

demographics, of University Hospital study, 57

Descartes, René, 49

detotalizing philosophy, of patient-centered care, 149

dialectical and analogical imagination rhetorical device, 183–184, *190*, *195*, 197

disappointing and baseless storytelling theme, *191*, 194

discomfort, in spirituality discussion, 94

discussion: on holistic care, 123; in pluralistic ignorance study, 110–112; in religious authority study, 83–84. *See also* spirituality discussion

Disenchantment of Secular Discourse, The (Smith), 221n6

distrust, of authority, 76–77

Durkheim, Emile, 25; on sacredness of individual, 19

efficiency, as social structure value, 6

Egyptian religions: on holistic health, 34, 44; on illness moralizing, 44

elective parochialism, Warner on, 210

emotionally alienating spiritualism, 139

emotionally authenticating spiritualism, 139

emotionally inconsequential spiritualism, 139

emotional well-being, of caregivers, 132

emotions: caritas through, 7, 29, 31, 206; in workplace, 122–124. *See also* spiritual meaning pathways

ethic of caritas, 38, 203–205; actor importance for, 206–207; Weber on, 208

ethics: Axial, 14–16, 221n5; Greek medicine medical, 45; justice and care rhetorical device, 183, 184–185, *190*, *195*; nurses spiritual care code of, 54; spiritual care styles puzzle of, 148–155; Weber on salvation religions loving and care, 17

Evans, John, 15

faith: compassion code of traditions of, 17; in goodness of humanity, 10; Weber on science conflict with, 19–20

faith-based hospitals, 34–35, 46–47

false consensus effect, 97–98

false uniqueness effect, 97–98

familial therapies, 164–165, *165*, *166*

Ferngren, Gary: on ancient religions, 43–44; on Greek medicine as science, 44

Frank, Arthur, 177

frontline staff: care of human spirit responsibility, 14, 24; COVID-19 patients and, 14; health care institutions perception from, 28; human suffering empathic connection, 16; narratives on science and spiritual care, 37; for secular medicine and spiritual dignity, 13

"Giving Up on God" (Inglehart), 207
Goffman, Erving, 148; identity theory, 154–155; on spiritual care, 146–147, 149, 168, 169
Greek medicine: Armstrong on, 45; body-soul analogy of, 44, 45, 49; compassionate understanding of suffering, 45; Ferngren on, 44; Hippocratic Oath, 45; medical ethics and, 45; nursing and, 51; as science, 34, 44–45, 223n2
group: in-group and out-group ignorance, 97; in-group morality, 216; worthiness of care and, 11

Habits of the Heart (Bellah), 23–24
Haidt, Jonathan, 13
harm-based morality, 216
health: biopsychosocial model of, 49, 50, 167; holistic models of, 34, 44, 50; social model of, 49–50
health care: frontline staff perception of institutions of, 28; movement spirituality, 35, 52–54; symbolic interactionist perspective on, 186–187
Hein v. FFRF, 54
Hippocratic Oath, 45
historical development, of caritas: almshouses and faith-based hospitals, 34–35; ancient religions on retributive misfortune, 34, 44; Christianity care to sick, 34; Egyptian and Mesopotamian religions on holistic health, 34, 44; Greek medicine as science, 34, 44–45, 223n2; spirituality in health care movement, 35, 52–54
holistic care, 50; at academic medical centers, 5; discussion on, 123; modern

care systems and, 12–13; spiritual care facet of, 10, 53
holistic health, 50; Egyptian and Mesopotamian religion on, 34, 44
horizontal dimension of religion, 10
horizontal relations, in negotiated orders, 129–130, 224n4
hospitals: caritas loose coupling in, 8; faith-based, 34–35, 46–47; objective, dispassionate criteria in, 12; optional spiritual care in, 54; PICU in, 111–112; public and poor, 47–48; rationalization core logic, 8; UPMC, 63–65, 87, 117; workers improvisation of spirituality in, 9. See also academic medical centers; Clinical Pastoral Education; University Hospital
HR. See human relations
human dignity: Weber on rationalization risk to, 21. See also spiritual dignity
humanitarianism, 23
humanity: Axial Age spiritual development of, 11; faith in goodness of, 10; Weber on spiritual foundation of shared, 16–17
humanity and sanctity restoration, 203–210; chief actors for, 211–212; defining problem for, 212; final thoughts on, 220; looking forward, 217–220; objections to, 214–217; rationalization conception, 212–213; religion characterization, 213–214
humanizing ideologies, in spiritual care styles, 155–156
human relations (HR) management model, 124–125
human spirit, teachers care responsibility, 14
human suffering: Axial Age on care opportunity from, 45; frontline staff empathic connection for, 16; Greek medicine compassionate understanding of, 45; rationalization and dehumanization of, 26; religions on positive role of, 45; scientific systems and, 4–5; spiritual concerns from, 4–5; spiritual understanding of,

37; television and Internet impact on, 25; Weber on, 182; Weber on caritas origins to deal with, 17; Western humanitarianism to alleviate, 23
humor, spirituality and, 218–219

ICN. *See* International Council of Nurses
identity: Goffman theory of, 154–155; meaning attached to roles, 154; practice perspectives and, 154–155
illness: ancient religions treatment of, 44; Egyptian and Mesopotamian religion moralizing of, 44; religion understanding of, 43–46
immunosuppression therapy, transplants and, 86–87
impersonal quality: of modern care systems, 15–16; Weber on rationalization, 120
individuals: Robinson on sacred mystery within, 15; Weber and Durkheim on sacredness of, 19
Inglehart, Ronald, 207
in-group: ignorance, 97; morality, 216
institutions: academic medical centers as rationalized, 30; frontline staff perception of health care, 28; negotiated orders involvement of outside, 131–132; spiritual care styles and total, 148–149; storytelling reflected in, *191*, 193
International Council of Nurses (ICN) Code of Ethics, 54
Internet, human suffering impacted by, 25
interpersonal networks, spirituality discussion and, 102, 108
interpersonal relations seminar (IRS), of CPE, 92, 118–119
Islam, Axial Age and, 45–46
issue prominence, spirituality discussion and, 102, 108

James, William, 113, 221n3
Jaspers, Karl: on Axial Age, 22; Weber and, 16–17

job work orientation, 159, 161, *162*, *165*, 225n5
Joint Commission: Mandate on Assessment of Spiritual Needs, 56; spirituality entry in 1999 standards of, 53
Journal of Christian Nursing, 53
Judaism, UPMC roots of, 117
Judeo-Christian concept: caritas as, 222n10; theological anthropocentrism and, 15
justice and care ethic rhetorical device, 183, 184–185, *190*, *195*

Kleinman, Arthur, 27

language: caritas through, 7, 29, 31, 206; comfort in spiritual, 94; Weber on shared, 93. *See also* spirituality discussion
lived religion perspective, 38, 209, *211*, 213, 225n2; shortcomings of, 181; on spirituality, 80; storytelling and, 179
loose coupling for caritas, in hospital, 8
love for all people. *See* caritas

Mandate on Assessment of Spiritual Needs, of Joint Commission, 56
Marx, Karl, 25
McClain, Colleen, 49
meaning: of caritas, 9; corporate-sponsored spiritual, 122–127; identity attached to roles, 154; of pluralistic ignorance, 94–95; of spirituality, 9–10, *135*, 135–138, *137*, 222n9; Weber on rationalization threat to, 20; Weber on workplace emotional displays and, 122, 123. *See also* spiritual meaning pathways
measures, for pluralistic ignorance study, 104–105
mechanical dehumanization, Christoff on negative consequences of, 16
Medicaid, academic medical centers and, 48
medical ethics, Greek medicine and, 45

medical research, at academic medical centers, 47

Medicare, 70; academic medical centers and, 48, 73

Merton, Robert, 99

Mesopotamian religion: on holistic health, 34, 44; on illness moralizing, 44

methods: in narrative styles study, 188–189; in religious authority study, 80–81; in spiritual care styles study, 158–159; in spiritual meaning pathways study, 133–134; in University Hospital study, 31–33

Middle Ages, nursing and religion association in, 51

military: mandatory spiritual care in, 54; spiritual governance in, 70, 85

Miller, Dale, 97

misperceptions: conjoint determinants in pluralistic ignorance study, *109*, 109–110; independent determinants in pluralistic ignorance study, 108, *108*

Mitroff, Ian, 77

models: biopsychosocial health, 49, 50, 167; culture of patient-centered, 152; HR management, 124–125; patient-centered, 28, 149, 152; social of health, 49–50

modern care systems: controversies over, 23; ethic of caritas in, 38, 203–207; holistic care in, 12–13; impersonal quality of, 15–16; objective, dispassionate criteria for, 12; patient-centered model, 28

modern society: caritas durability in, 38; Weber on religion social construction in, 10

moral dilemmas, of caregivers, 25

moral engineer *vs.* moral bricoleur spiritual care style, *157*, 157–158

morality, harm-based and in-group, 216

moral omnivore *vs.* moral univore spiritual care style, 156–157, *157*

movements: Axial Age religious, 11; spirituality in health care, 35, 52–54

mutual observability, pluralistic ignorance and high, 99–100

narrative: caritas through, 7, 29, 31, 206. *See also* storytelling

narrative medicine, 180; shortcomings of, 181–182

narrative styles study, 187; conclusion, 199–201; methods, 188–189; spirituality and medical science compatibility, 9, 198–199; storyteller attributes and circumstances reflections, 198; story themes, 189–191, *190*, *191*

Nash, Laura, 77

negotiated orders of hospital cultures, 133; caregiver emotional well-being, 132; cognitive frames, 130–131; horizontal relations, 129–130, 224n4; outside institutions involvement, 131–132; vertical relations, 128–129

New Age therapies, 152, 156, 164, 165, 166, *166*

Nightingale, Florence, 51–52

nurses: colleague conversations about spirituality, 36–37; common spiritual care practices, 37; human element of clinical practice, 50; missing opinions and experiences of, 55; Nightingale as, 51–52; opinions on becoming surrogate chaplains, 81–84; patient spiritual concerns about dying and, 53; patient spiritual well-being care, 5; pluralistic ignorance application to, 102–103; religious authority of, 71; scientific systems training, 5; spiritual care opinions, *81*, 81–82; on spirituality and medical science compatibility, 5, 9, 37, 198–199; spirituality defined by, 56

nursing: alternative therapies and, 53; code of ethics on spiritual care by, 54; Greek medicine and, 51; Middle Ages religion association with, 51; practices as spiritual, 37; religion historical roots of, 29, 51; religious affiliations of schools of, 51; scientific credentials emphasis, 52; spiritual care and,

50–56; spirituality and scholarship of, 54–55

objectivity, as social structure value, 6
"On a Certain Blindness in Human Beings" (James), 113
opinions, of nurses: on becoming surrogate chaplains, 81–84; missing experiences and, 55; spiritual care, *81*, 81–82; University Hospital spirituality in health care, 56–62
organizational expressions, of caritas, 46–48
organizational phenomenon, of spirituality, 31–32
out-group ignorance, 97
outside institutions involvement, in negotiated orders, 132

pathology, biomedicine focus on, 49
patient-centered model: culture of, 152; detotalizing philosophy of, 149; of modern care systems, 28. *See also* holistic care
patients: nurses and spiritual concerns about dying, 53; spiritual care and satisfaction of, 223n5
pediatric intensive care unit (PICU), 111–112
Persians, The (Aeschylus), 56
person-centered approach to care, 53–54
perspectives: care-centered, 214; caritas-centered, 38, 213; caritas neglect by secularization, 209–210; health care symbolic interactionist, 186–187; identity and practice, 154–155; lived religion, 38, 80, 179, 181, 209, *211*, 213, 225n2; secularization, 38, 179, 209–210, *211*, 212–213
philosophical anthropocentrism, of Singer, 15
physical proximity: pluralistic ignorance and, 100–101; spirituality discussion and, 100–101
PICU. *See* pediatric intensive care unit
pluralistic ignorance, 223n1; absolute, 97; Allport on, 98; application to nurses,

102–103; cultures of organizations and, 101; high mutual observability and, 99–100; meaning of, 94–95; Merton on, 99; nature of, 97–98; past research on, 98–100; physical proximity and, 100–101; Prentice and Miller on, 97; relative, 97; sources of, 101–102; speech norms and, 101; spirituality discussion relevance, 95–97; in workplace, 102
pluralistic ignorance study: conclusion, 112–116; data on, 103; discussion, 110–112; measures for, 104–105; misperceptions conjoint determinants, *109*, 109–110; misperceptions independent determinants, 108, *108*; PICU and, 111–112; preliminary findings, 105–107, *106*, *107*
population, in University Hospital study, 29–30, 222n13
poverty: academic medical centers and, 47–48; Marx on capitalism and, 25
preliminary findings, in pluralistic ignorance study, 105–107, *106*, *107*
Prentice, Deborah, 97
prisons, spiritual governance in, 70, 85
professionalism, care for strangers and, 149–151
professions, religious authority disappearing boundaries, 78–79
pro-spirituality, in University Hospital study, 57–58
public funding, of academic medical centers, 30, 48
public religion, 208; through care for strangers, 6–7; Weber care-centered, 7

Rabbinic Judaism, Axial Age and, 45–46
rationalization: Brooks on human needs, 14–15; competing value systems and, 18; conception of humanity and sanctity restoration, 212–213; history of conflict between caritas and, 11–12; hospitals core logic of, 8; human suffering dehumanization from, 26; spiritual care styles and, *155*; spiritual

rationalization (*continued*)
human qualities extinguished by, 18;
Weber on caritas threat from, 7, 18–19,
209, 220; Weber on human dignity
risk from, 21; Weber on impersonal
quality of, 120; Weber on meaning
threat from, 20; Weber on unexpected
harm from, 18–19
rationalized institution, academic
medical centers as, 30
reenchantment, through storytelling,
177–178
reflected in institutions and practices
storytelling theme, *191*, 193
reflexive spirituality discussion, 100
relative pluralistic ignorance, 97
religion: ancient, 34, 43–44; care
for stranger as value of, 5, 8, 13;
characterization of humanity and
sanctity restoration, 213–214; decline
in, 223n3; horizontal compared
to vertical dimensions of, 10; on
human suffering positive role, 45;
illness understanding by, 43–46;
James on personal, 221n3; lived
religion perspective, 38, 80, 179,
181, 209, *211*, 213, 225n2; Middle
Ages nursing affiliation with, 51;
nursing historical roots in, 29,
51; person-giving power of, 8;
presence-enhancing power of, 7; as
private matter, 23–24; secularization
perspective of, 38, 179, 209–210, *211*,
212–213; Sullivan on naturalization
of, 54; Weber on modern society
social construction of, 10; Weber on
salvation, 17
religious authority: continuing relevance
of, 79–80; craft-based versions of,
71, 78–80, 86; evidence of declining,
75–76; literature on secularization
and, 71; of nurses, 71; professions
disappearing boundaries, 78–79;
scholarship on secularization, 74–75;
secularization declining, 75; at
University Hospital, 73–74; Weber
understanding of, 66, 71

religious authority study: conclusion of,
84–86; discussion on, 83–84; methods,
80–81; nurses on becoming surrogate
chaplains, 81–82
religious etiquette, spirituality discussion
and, 96
religious movements, in Axial Age, 11
religious therapies, 164–165, *166*
research: academic medical centers
medical, 47; literature on spiritual
storytelling, 179–183; narrative styles
study, 187–201, *190*, *191*; pluralistic
ignorance past, 98–100; pluralistic
ignorance study, 103–116, *106*,
107, *108*, *109*; religious authority
and secularization literature, 71;
religious authority study, 80–86;
secularization scholarship, 74–75;
spiritual care styles study, 158–170,
160, *161*, *162*, *163*, *164*, *165*, *166*;
spiritual meaning pathways study,
133–140, *135*, *137*. *See also* University
Hospital study
retributive misfortune, ancient religions
on, 34, 44
revealed through events and transitions
storytelling theme, *191*, 192–193
rhetorical devices and narrative style,
178–179; Aristotle and, 183; centripetal
and centrifugal framings, 183, 184,
190, *195–197*; combinations of,
194–198; dialectical and analogical
imagination, 183–184, *190*, *195*, 197;
justice and care ethics, 183, 184–185,
190, *195*; reflections on, 185; sacrificial
and expressive self, 182, 185, *190*, *195*,
197
Robinson, Marilynne, 15
Rogerian therapy approach, of chaplains,
69, 92, 119, 144
Rosenfeld, Barry, 49

sacralization, 77, 82, 86
sacrificial and expressive self rhetorical
device, 182, 185, *190*, *195*, *197*
salvation religions, Weber on ethic of
loving and care, 17

science: frontline staff narratives
on spiritual care and, 37; Greek
medicine as, 34, 44–45, 223n2; nurses
on spirituality compatibility with
medical, 5, 9, 37, 198–199; Weber on
conflict between faith and, 19–20
"Science as Vocation" lecture, of Weber,
176
scientific systems: nurse training in, 5;
spiritual concerns trivialized by, 5;
suffering and, 4–5; Weber on, 19–22
scientific vocations, Weber on, 19–22
secularization: countertrends in, 76–78;
religious authority and decline in, 75;
religious authority and literature on,
71; scholarship on, 74–75; as social
structure value, 6; Weber on, 35
secularization perspective, 38, 211,
212–213; caritas neglect by, 209–210;
storytelling and, 179
Singer, Peter, 15
Smith, Steven, 221n6
social justice, 42
social model of health, 49–50
social science, Weber on universal
happiness and, 21–22
social structure values, of efficiency,
objectivity, secularization, 6
sociology, value-neutral approach of, 26
sociotechnical conditions, spirituality
discussion and, 102, 108
Soul of Care, The (Kleinman), 27
speech norms, pluralistic ignorance and,
101
spiritual but not religious caregivers, 24
spiritual care, 225n2; faith in goodness
of humanity and, 10; Goffman on,
146–147, 149, 168, 169; holistic, 10,
53; hospital optional, 54; military
mandatory, 54; nurse common
practices of, 37; nurse opinions on, 81,
81–82; nursing and, 50–56; in nursing
code of ethics, 54; responsibility of,
35–36
spiritual care styles: care for self, 155;
caregiving and professionalism,
150–151; chaplain intern experience,

143–145; developments in, 153–154;
ethical puzzle of, 148–155; humanizing
ideologies, 155–156; identity and
practice perspectives, 154–155;
moral engineer vs. moral bricoleur,
157, 157–158; moral omnivore
vs. moral univore, 156–157, 157;
rationalization, 155; total institutions
and dignity challenge, 148–149;
transplant experience, 170–172; work
orientations practical implications,
151–152
spiritual care styles study: conclusion,
166–170; intervention circumstances,
162–163, 163; methods, 158–159; spiritual
therapies, 163–166, 164, 165, 166; work
orientations, 159–162, 160, 161, 162
spiritual concerns: from human suffering,
4–5; scientific systems trivialization
of, 5
spiritual dignity: Axial Age advocacy
for, 5, 11–12; frontline staff for secular
medicine and, 13; total institutions
challenge for, 148–149
spiritual dimension, of caritas, 9, 203,
222n10
spiritual governance, in prisons and
military, 70, 85
spiritualism: emotionally alienating,
139; emotionally authenticating, 139;
emotionally inconsequential, 139
spirituality: academic medical centers
incorporation of, 30; being human
and, 221n6; biomedicine and, 49;
in health care movement, 35, 52–54;
hospital workers improvisation
of, 8; humor and, 218–219; Joint
Commission 1999 standards entry on,
53; lived religion perspective on, 80;
meaning of, 9–10, 135, 135–138, 137,
222n9; nurse colleague conversations
about, 36–37; nurse definition of,
56; nursing scholarship on, 54–55; as
organizational phenomenon, 31–32;
through storytelling, 173–202; talk
avoidance about, 36; transcendent
quality of, 10, 178, 221n4, 222n7;

spirituality (*continued*)
University Hospital on, 9; University
Hospital study on efficacy and
inclusivity of, 60–62, *61*; University
Hospital study on promotion of,
58–60, *59*; University Hospital study
operationalization of, 30–31; in
workplace, 77–78, 126, 223n2
spirituality and healing, international
conference at University Hospital, 30
spirituality discussion: chaplain intern
experience and, 90–93; discomfort
in, 94; interpersonal networks and,
102, 108; issue prominence and, 102,
108; physical proximity and, 100–101;
pluralistic ignorance and, 94–116;
pluralistic ignorance relevance
to, 95–97; reflexive, 100; religious
etiquette and, 96; sociotechnical
conditions and, 102, 108; transplant
experience, 116–117
spiritual love. See *agape*; *ahaba*
spiritual meaning pathways: authenticity
and, 120–121, 125, 133–134; chaplain
intern experience and, 118–120;
corporate-sponsored, 122–127; hospital
cultures as negotiated orders, 128–133;
transplant experience, 140–142
spiritual meaning pathways study:
conclusion, 139–140; emotional
consequences, 138–139; methods,
133–134; preliminary findings, 134–135;
work culture combined effects, 136–
138, *137*; work culture direct effects,
135, 135–136
spiritual understandings, through
storytelling, 186–187
storytelling: chaplain intern
experience and, 173–176; Frank
on disenchantment and, 177;
literature on spiritual, 179–183;
lived religion perspective and, 179;
reenchantment through, 177–178;
secularization perspective and, 179;
spirituality through, 173–202; spiritual
understandings through, 186–187;
transplant experience and, 201–202.

See also rhetorical devices and
narrative style
storytelling themes on spirituality,
189–191, *190*; bound in relationships,
191, 192; disappointing and baseless,
191, 194; reflected in institutions
and practices, *191*, 193; revealed
through events and transitions, *191*,
192–193; subject to constraints and
uncertainties, *191*, 193
subject to constraints and uncertainties
storytelling theme, *191*, 193
suffering. See human suffering
Sullivan, Winnifred Fallers, 54
symbolic interactionist perspective, of
health care, 186–187

teachers, human spirit care
responsibility, 14
teaching hospitals. See academic medical
centers
television, human suffering impacted
by, 25
therapy: familial, 164–165, *165*, *166*;
New Age, 152, 156, 164, 165, 166, *166*;
nursing alternative, 53; religious,
164–165, *166*; Rogerian approach of
chaplains, 69, 92, 119, 144; spiritual
care styles study on spiritual, 163–
166, *164*, *165*, *166*; transplants and
immunosuppression, 86–87
total institutions, in spiritual care styles,
148–149
transcendent quality, of spirituality, 10,
178, 221n4, 222n7
transplant experience, 1–4, 62, 66, 89;
immunosuppression therapy, 86–87;
spiritual care styles and, 170–172;
spirituality discussion and, 116–117;
spiritual meaning pathways and, 140–
142; storytelling and, 201–202; testing
for, 87–88; UPMC and, 63–65, 87, 117

universal happiness, Weber on social
science and, 21–22
University Hospital: chaplains program
termination, 71, 74, 85, 204; religious

authority at, 73–74; on spirituality, 9; spirituality and healing international conference, 30; spirituality in health care opinions, 56–62

University Hospital study: analytical and personal combination, 32–33; contributions to, 33–34; demographics of, 57; methods, 31–33; on nurse pro-spirituality, 57–58; nurse surveys and interviews at, 5, 222n13; opinions on spirituality promotion, 58–60, 59; population, 29–30, 222n13; on spiritual conceptions, 57, 58; on spirituality as organizational phenomenon, 31–32; on spirituality efficacy and inclusivity, 60–62, 61; spirituality operationalization, 30–31. *See also* narrative styles study; pluralistic ignorance study; religious authority study; spiritual care styles study; spiritual meaning pathways study

University of Pittsburgh Medical Center (UPMC): Judaism roots of, 117; organ transplant center at, 63–65, 87

value-neutral approach, of sociology, 26
values: care for stranger as religion, 5, 8, 13; efficiency as social structure, 6; objectivity as social structure, 6; rationalization and competing systems of, 18; secularization as social structure, 6; Weber on rationality of, 212

vertical dimension of religion, 10
vertical relations, in negotiated orders, 128–129

Veteran's Administration, spiritual governance in, 70, 85

Warner, Stephen, 210
Weber, Max, 24–28, 56; on brotherliness, 17, 222n10; care-centered public religion, 7; on caritas routine action, 37; on culture, 30–31; on ethic of caritas, 208; on fate of caritas and, 22–24; on human suffering, 182; on human suffering and caritas origins, 17; on impersonal quality of

rationalization, 120; Jaspers and, 16–17; private life of, 22; on rationalization threat to caritas, 7, 18–19, 209, 220; religious authority understanding, 66, 71; on sacredness of individual, 19; on science and faith conflict, 19–20; on scientific vocations, 19–22; on secularization, 35; on shared humanity spiritual foundation, 16–17; on shared language, 93; on social action, 146; on social construction of religion in modern society, 10; on social science and universal happiness, 21–22; on unexpected harm from rationalization, 18–19; on value rationality, 212; on workplace meaning and emotional displays, 122, 123; on world disenchantment, 41–42, 176–177

Western humanitarianism: human suffering alleviation and, 23; self-serving justification for intervention, 23

work culture: spiritual meaning combined effects, 136–138, 137; spiritual meaning direct effects, 135, 135–136

work orientations: of calling, 159, 161–162, 162, 163, 164, 165, 166, 169, 225n5, 225n7; of career, 159, 161, 162, 163, 164, 165, 166, 225n5, 225n7; familial therapies, 164–165, 165, 166; of job, 159, 161, 162, 165, 225n5; New Age therapies, 152, 156, 164, 165, 166, 166; religious therapies, 164–165, 166; spiritual care practical implications, 151–152; spiritual care styles study on, 159–162, 160, 161, 162

workplace: Abbott on, 78; academic medical centers overburdened, 84; emotions in, 122–124; Nash and Mitroff on spirituality in, 77; pluralistic ignorance in, 102; publications on spirituality in, 78; spirituality in, 77–78, 126, 223n2; Weber on meaning and emotional displays in, 122, 123

world disenchantment, Weber on, 41–42, 176–177

.

GPSR Authorized Representative: Easy Access System Europe, Mustamäe tee 50, 10621 Tallinn, Estonia, gpsr.requests@easproject.com